love you so much
a shared memoir

To Linda,
who was so kind and
welcoming to my mother.
Cherish every day!
Karen Anne Young

love you so much

a shared memoir

Victoria Zacheis Greve
& Karen Greve Young

SUMMERTIME PUBLISHING

First Published Great Britain 2011
by Summertime Publishing

ISBN 978-1-904881-36-0

Design by Hilary Hanson Bruel
www.hansonbrueldesign.com

This book is dedicated to GG's grandchildren

Jeffrey and Kathryn
&
Andrew and Adam

CONTENTS

love you so much

a shared memoir

INTRODUCTION
December 30, 2002

KAREN

In my mind, I've done this hundreds of times over the past month: written the first line, and then full paragraphs, pages, and chapters. I've discovered that I am a brilliant mental writer during my commute on the London underground, while cooking dinner, and especially in bed — before going to sleep, upon waking up in the morning, and during those countless times I awaken during the night, anxious about what this book means and how it will unfold.

Mom and I hope that writing our story will be a shared cathartic experience for us, while raising awareness of ovarian cancer's nearly silent symptoms and helping other women and their families cope with the disease.

This won't be easy. For our story to have merit, we will need to be ruthlessly honest in portraying what we remember from the past three years. A sugar-coated tale in which the only disappointments, setbacks and frustrations are medical will not serve our purpose. Of course, most of the disappointments, setbacks, and frustrations have been medical, but not all.

Cancer has a way of recreating relationships, shifting the important people in our lives into new roles or strengthening bonds already there. Some transformations — those people who went from being good friends to providing emotional life support — will be easy subjects. The negative transformations will be harder to write about accurately — it is those that I fear, but that will be the most rewarding to us and to our audience if we can keep ourselves honest. And I believe that we can.

We are writing this for ourselves and for our incredible network of family and friends who have supported us during her illness. We are also writing it for the 225,000 women who are diagnosed with ovarian cancer each year, two-thirds of whom are diagnosed at advanced stages of disease. We are especially writing it in memory of the 140,000 women annually who lose the battle with ovarian cancer.[1]

One of the most frustrating aspects of our experience has been the utter lack of awareness of ovarian cancer in our society. It is often called "the silent killer" because its symptoms — persistent episodes of bloating, pelvic or abdominal pain, urinary urgency or frequency, and difficulty eating or feeling full quickly — are not widely recognized or understood. My mother had every early-stage symptom of ovarian cancer for several months before massive abdominal swelling finally led to her advanced-stage diagnosis. She had no idea that her fatigue and digestive issues

---

[1] Worldwide incidence and mortality data retrieved on May 26, 2011, from http://globocan.iarc.fr/. U.S. diagnosis stage data retrieved on May 26, 2011, from http://www.seer.cancer.gov/statfacts/html/ovary.html.

were the first symptoms of an insidious disease at work in her body.

Since her diagnosis, my mother's cancer has been beaten back by surgery and many chemotherapy regimens, but it still persists. Her gorgeous short hair with its thick salt and pepper waves has been ravaged by chemotherapy and replaced by wigs and hats, growing back curlier, and with increasing salt to pepper.

Meanwhile, our lives continue, lived through the lens of cancer patient and cancer patient's daughter. Our life events, daily activities, and relationships, punctuated by medical appointments and decisions, comprise the fabric of this book. This is my mother's story, and mine.

Neither of us is rich or famous. We are just women, writing about our shared experience. We hope that this book will help to drive awareness of ovarian cancer among other women and families. We dream that awareness will drive demand for more information and support for increased funding of research into ovarian cancer prevention, screening, and treatments that will save women's lives.

Now, it's time for our story to begin.

BEFORE
Spring and Summer 1999

VICKI

It's a wonderful thing to be healthy. Although I had bouts of illness as a child, I've spent my entire adult life as a strong, healthy person. My husband, Cliff, and I have been extremely conscientious about taking lots of vitamins, maintaining a healthy diet, and getting adequate sleep and regular checkups. We make every effort to keep up our exercise routines. Except for the occasional cold and those relentless extra few pounds, we are in good shape. So I never expected to get cancer.

One chronic problem both of us have is the continuing fight to maintain a "good" weight. In February 1999, my weight reached an all-time high of 170 pounds, which is way too heavy for my five foot seven-inch frame. I was beginning to feel like I was carrying around a ton every time I went upstairs and had less energy than I needed. I had tried to diet before without much success. But this time I was determined, and with a healthy diet I managed to drop 15 pounds by June.

To celebrate my success, my daughter, Karen, and I treated ourselves to a week at Canyon Ranch spa in Tucson, Arizona. There, I would certainly begin an exercise regimen that would firm up my sagging skin and muscles and help me lose another 15 pounds to achieve a weight of 140 before Christmas.

Canyon Ranch was my first experience at a spa and I loved it. The food was delicious and appetizing. I even learned a few things about improving meals at home. The classes were arranged in a way that I could pace myself and sample a variety of different techniques — yoga, tai chi, pilates, cycling, weights, and aerobics — the list was endless. We also went on a beautiful, albeit exhausting hike in the hilly Arizona desert.

KAREN

One of the highlights of our week in Tucson was a fitness hike in the Sonoran Desert. We'd chosen a moderate hike — a two-mile trek uphill followed by lunch and the return trip down. The two women guiding the hike looked like they exercised twelve hours a day in the desert sun. One guide led, followed by Mom, me, two other guests, and then the second guide.

We started off at an easy pace, probably about two and a half miles an hour. As we wound up the desert path, surrounded by Saguaro cacti and sagebrush, my mom kept practically on the heels of the guide. The guide responded by increasing the pace. Within a few minutes, ten yards separated us from the three hikers in back. Soon, they were out of sight as we cruised up the path at a rapid clip, my mom just behind the guide while I followed a few paces behind.

After a mile, our guide asked if we wanted to stop for water. "I thought you'd never ask," was Mom's labored response. Her face was red and she was breathing heavily — no surprise given our pace.

As we drank, she hesitantly asked if our pace was typical for this hike.

"Not at all," the guide replied. "This pace is much more rigorous than we usually do, but we try to cater each hike to the fitness level of the guests. The way you were on my heels, I thought you wanted to walk faster."

Mom was stunned. "You mean it was my fault that we did that pace?"

"No, it was great!" was the guide's enthusiastic reply. "You were really pushing it. We can take it slower the rest of the way up, though, if you'd prefer."

She gratefully agreed and we resumed our ascent. We started out at a slower pace, but Mom kept pushing on the heels of the guide. To the guide's credit, she controlled our speed by stopping to show us particular flora, and to point out the occasional lizard skirting across the path. Still, lunch at the top was a welcome respite.

I laughed at my mother.

"The way you were pushing us up the mountain, it was like you were trying out for the Olympic hiking team!"

She sounded frustrated when she replied. "I've always had that problem — always pushing too hard and not knowing when to take it easy."

"It's not a problem," I insisted. "It's one of the things I admire about you. Though I worry sometimes, because you don't really pay attention to your limits."

"Limits, what limits?" Mom quipped. No wonder I tried to emulate her energy and spirit.

VICKI

When I got home from Tucson, I was sure I would have a wonderful surprise on the scale. Unfortunately, the surprise was that I hadn't lost an ounce. After a week at the spa, I was more determined than ever to continue the weight loss regimen I had started earlier in the year, through diet and exercise.

By profession, I was a Certified Public Accountant working in KPMG's exempt organization tax practice. November 15th was a huge tax deadline for my clients. Between client meetings and reviewing tax returns, I had barely a few minutes each day to do anything except work, eat, and sleep. My exercising became spotty at best.

Then, as a result of trying to fit the treadmill into a small amount of time, I was careless about stretching and pacing myself and I developed a stress fracture in my right fibia. The orthopedist gave me a stiff boot to wear to protect the bone from further damage and prescribed crutches. Just what I needed while I was trying to deal with everything else! In the meantime, my husband Cliff had severed a nerve in his left thumb while cutting vegetables for dinner, requiring microscopic surgery and many weeks of healing. What a decrepit pair we had become! Little did I know that this was only the beginning of more serious health issues.

Although I kept careful watch on my food intake, without the treadmill my weight started to climb again. By the end of September I was back up to 160! Did I need to do more stringent dieting? I felt exhausted all the time, but I attributed that to my demands at the office.

Early in October, I had my regular check up with my gynecologist. I had been going to him since I was pregnant with Karen in 1973. I mentioned my recent issues with intestinal gas and constipation. Neither one is very easy to discuss, but both had to be brought under control because they were uncomfortable and could be embarrassing at work. He suggested that I try to change my diet to exclude yogurt and other things that were known to cause upset stomach. If that didn't work, he would recommend a gastroenterologist. I was also extremely tired — just like every other 54-year-old woman I knew.

In the middle of October, my weight really began climbing, sometimes as much as a pound a day. On the 30th, we went to my sister's annual Halloween party and I had to wear one of my only two dresses that didn't have a waist-line because my waist had gotten completely out of control. I could no longer button or zip my slacks and everything with a waistline was uncomfortably tight. At this point, I began to suspect that my extreme fatigue wasn't just related to job stress.

I felt terrible, with intestinal gas and bloating. I decided to go to the internist because I was sure this wasn't a female problem that my gynecologist should address. The first appointment I could get was two days away.

KAREN

I had moved to San Francisco after college, lured by a high-tech investment bank. The hours were grueling; it wasn't unusual for me to finally leave the office in the early morning as others were arriving to start their day. When I wasn't working insane hours to position myself for business school, I ran countless miles along the San Francisco Bay and Pacific Ocean. I ran my first marathon in 1997, quickly followed by three others.

My hard work at the office paid off and I started at Stanford's Graduate School of Business (GSB) that fall. It was heaven for me as an avid marathoner and aspiring triathlete. There were miles of running trails, including the locally infamous "Dish" — a network of hilly trails in parkland surrounding several Stanford satellite dishes — and the four mile campus loop. As a student, I also had access to two 50-meter, perfectly regulated, outdoor swimming pools that were available for recreational lap swimming between varsity swimming and water polo practices.

Of course, I wasn't at Stanford for the athletic facilities. The pinnacle among many high points of my experience at Stanford was my fellow students. I was amazed at the breadth of exposure and accomplishments that came up in casual and classroom conversations among my 360 classmates. The common threads linking nearly everyone were energy, talent, drive, ambition, and enthusiasm for the GSB experience. At any given hour of any day, it was easy to find a person or group to join for a hike or run, dinner out, shooting pool at a local bar, dancing at a San Francisco club, or nearly anything else. I had never in my life been nearly as social as I was in my first fall at the GSB — and it was all justified as "networking".

My roommate, Sarah, and I became friends immediately based on our many similarities, not least of which was that we were both tall, athletic women who loved to run for miles and miles, and then undo our fitness with frozen margaritas rimmed with salt. We traded stories and experiences while hanging out in her room or mine, traipsing back and forth through the shared kitchen that linked our bright yellow bedrooms.

In one of these conversations, I confessed to her that I

was interested in dating one of our classmates, Geordie.

I met Geordie at a party the week before school started. We were introduced by a mutual friend from Harvard College, where we'd overlapped for three years without ever meeting. Coincidentally, Geordie and I had every class together that first quarter at Stanford. I discovered that he was a Canadian ice hockey and rugby player who'd completed an Ironman triathlon and graduated *summa cum laude* in astrophysics from Harvard. I soon found myself scanning campus for him whenever I was out. He was easy to spot — at six feet tall, he had a broad, powerful back and arms; short, straight dark hair framed his square, chiseled face and green eyes. Ruggedly handsome, his only blight seemed to be that he cared little for appearances, wearing a ragged t-shirt or Harvard varsity sweatshirt with khaki shorts and sandals every single day to class.

By late October, my crush on Geordie had grown and I was rapidly losing my resolve not to date anyone until at least Christmas. I still had no idea if he was interested, but I knew for sure that I was. On the 30th, I went to the GSB Halloween Party with Sarah and other friends. The party was held at a derelict Silicon Valley mansion known as the "Halloween House" for the party thrown annually by its GSB tenants. Empowered by my disguise as Betty Boop, I had a long conversation with Canuck Smurf and realized that my attraction was matched by the blue-faced, hockey stick-wielding Geordie.

The next morning, I couldn't wait to call Mom to tell her about my evening and the incredible guy I'd kissed. After telling her all about Geordie, I finally asked how things were at home and if she was excited for the arrival of trick-or-treaters.

She wasn't excited; she felt bloated and miserable. I vaguely remembered her mentioning it the week before, but had been so absorbed with my life at school that I hadn't really focused on it. As she told me about her discomfort on a drive with Dad into the country to see the fall foliage — which she usually loved doing — and her decision not to greet the trick-or-treaters that night, I started to worry. This was the first time that I realized that maybe her weight issues could be more than normal water retention or hormones.

DIAGNOSIS
October – November 1999

VICKI

Fortunately, my internist was only a block away from the office so walking over there with my crutches was relatively easy. I had been going to him for several years, primarily to address a slight elevation in blood pressure due to a variety of medications for depression (and maybe job stress). I felt silly going to him with my symptoms of being overweight and having bloating, fatigue, and intestinal gas. But he took my symptoms seriously. After a lengthy examination, he referred me to a gastroenterologist for further diagnosis.

Over the course of the next ten days, I had extensive testing, including x-rays, blood tests, and sonograms, most of them in the same building as my internist's office. In the meantime, the bloating got so bad that I couldn't button any of my skirts or pants. One evening, I went shopping for jumpers to wear to work. I had no idea what was wrong, but until I found out, I needed to be presentable at the office.

During this time, Cliff stepped on an acorn while raking leaves and fell on the sidewalk, breaking his right wrist. Now we were really a pair! He couldn't drive his stick shift Saturn because his right hand was in a cast, his left thumb having finally healed from his kitchen accident. I couldn't drive it either, because I couldn't handle the brake and clutch routine with my right leg's stress fracture. So we "shared" my Lexus. That meant that he dropped me off at the office in the morning on his way to work and picked me up late in the day.

On the day of my sonogram, Cliff dropped me off at my internist's office with a kiss and reminder to call him if I needed him. I was thinking I needed him to go to the sonogram with me, but didn't ask because he was busy with his work too. I didn't want to burden him by asking him to just sit with me during my tests.

However, the sonogram didn't turn out to be routine. When it was over, the technician told me to go upstairs to the doctor's office so that he could discuss the findings with me. So I went up on my crutches and was in his waiting room for only a few minutes before going in to see him.

The doctor looked serious and caring. He said the sonogram showed some involvement with my ovaries, and asked if I had seen my gynecologist recently. I described my appointment in October. My internist said I needed to see him again right away, because a gynecologist was the best person to handle my problems. I just sat there while the tears formed. I was stunned. He made the call for me and explained that it was urgent that I see the gynecologist, who agreed to wait for me although his office typically closed at noon on Friday. I thanked my internist and left.

I struggled with the tears all the way to the pay phone in the building. I would have to take a cab because I didn't have a car. I called Cliff to ask him to meet me at the gynecologist's, but I couldn't reach him by phone. So I left a message. I do a lot of that. He is very busy.

Then I called our son, Drew, who was living with us while he finished his Masters degree in Psychology. Fortunately his graduate school schedule included flexible hours, which he spent mostly at home studying. He agreed to meet me at the gynecologist's office. We both sat there while my internist and gynecologist discussed my situation on the phone.

I will be forever grateful to Drew for just being there for me. It must have been difficult for him, age 24, to be supporting his mother in this way.

My gynecologist hadn't done a CA-125 blood test in October, but he drew blood for one now. I was only vaguely aware that it was the test for a protein marker associated with ovarian cancer. The results wouldn't be available for several days. He also performed another sonogram. Then, Drew took me home and I spent the weekend just getting bigger and more uncomfortable. By now I weighed almost 170 pounds again.

KAREN

In the two weeks after Halloween, I talked to my parents even more than usual, which meant at least once a day. It seemed that Mom had different doctor's appointments or testing almost daily, and we were on an emotional roller coaster while she went from one to the next. I tried to say the "right" thing on the phone, but what is the right thing to say when your mother is going through a battery of tests and appointments to diagnose a mystery illness? We were hoping for the best while fearing the worst — and not knowing what the worst meant.

I had just come in from a run around the "Dish" one afternoon when Mom called to tell me about her doctor's appointment that morning. As she told me his comments about "involvement with her ovaries" and "appointment to biopsy the fluid sample," I couldn't really comprehend what she was saying. I kept asking questions that she and Dad couldn't answer.

I tried to hold myself together on the phone, but as soon as I hung up, I just sat at my desk and cried. After a few minutes, I heard Sarah's door open and close. I walked through the kitchen and knocked on her door.

"Hey, do you have a minute?"

"Of course." Then she saw my tears. "Oh my God, Karen. What's wrong? Come here."

I sank onto her bed and started to talk, then I hesitated. Sarah had lost her mother three years earlier from a complication with a routine knee surgery. Soon after, her father was diagnosed with pancreatic cancer. So far, he was fighting the cancer successfully with chemotherapy, but I knew that it weighed constantly on her mind. And I knew how desperately she missed her mother.

Regardless, she was my best friend at school and I needed a friend.

"I just got off the phone with my parents. The doctors don't know what's wrong with my mom. They said something about involvement with her ovaries, and they took a blood test for cancer." I dissolved into tears.

Sarah was my rock over the next few days. She managed to be there for me every time I needed to talk without ever pressuring me or imposing. I wasn't prepared to talk about Mom with our other classmates yet. It was all much too raw.

VICKI

On Tuesday afternoon, November 9th, my gynecologist made arrangements for me to go to a nearby hospital to have fluid removed from my abdomen. He said they might keep me there and do a hysterectomy so I should plan for that. It didn't occur to me that I might want to do a little research about the surgeon or solicit a second opinion. This whole issue seemed like an emergency situation.

The timing was just awful from a business perspective. Randy, the partner I worked for, came to my office for a debriefing on the dozens of tax returns and other projects that had November 15th deadlines. I had been concerned about making the deadlines even with overtime. Randy now faced the possibility of doing it for me without the familiarity I had with all the details. We were both stunned, but very professional.

Maybe the overwhelming workload kept me from dwelling on the severity of my illness. After all, the C word hadn't yet been uttered to me. I left a message on my voicemail saying that I would be out of the office for an undetermined period of time, telling callers to contact Randy directly. I had no time to alert the auditors or tax staff or clients that I would be out of the office, or why.

Because Cliff was working thirty minutes away in Virginia and I was in downtown Washington, DC, we met at the hospital. At least he was available to go with me. I took a cab to the local hospital's cancer center and started tearing up as I arrived. I wished it had been called something else, anything else, except a cancer center. After all, we weren't sure I had cancer, so I resented having to be treated at a cancer center. I checked in and met Cliff in the waiting room. We didn't wait very long. I remember saying to the first nurse I saw that I hoped I wouldn't be back again.

The oncology nurse coordinator spent the most time with us. We asked about my CA-125 result. She said that it was 1200. I had no frame of reference, so I asked her what was normal. Her response was that 10 or less was ideal, but under 35 was acceptable. Cliff asked what their diagnosis was. She said the working diagnosis was ovarian cancer, probably stage III because it seemed to have metastasized to other organs. They weren't sure yet which other organs, but it looked like the right kidney was involved.

So, the diagnosis was cancer, but I wasn't sure I believed it. How could I get cancer when no one in my family had ever had it? Besides, I was sure I was meant to live lots longer than my 54 years.

The fluid removal was a terrible experience. Cliff stood by the table the whole time while I was hooked up to monitors and a technician stuck a tube in my abdomen to suck out almost four liters of ugly brown fluid. The fluid tested benign. No cancer there. Thank goodness. I was hanging on to any hopeful sign I could find. I didn't like being sick and had no time for cancer. I went home, relieved that I wouldn't have to have a hysterectomy — at least not right away.

The next day at the office, I discussed with Randy the possible severity of my illness — yes, including the C word. He expressed such sensitivity and concern that I appreciated all the more that I worked for a man like him.

Cliff was able to take me for my colonoscopy and endoscopy, as well as my second fluid removal (four liters again!) but I was on my own for the rest of the appointments. Fortunately I had a great chauffeur in Drew, who was such a good sport about driving me.

The day I met with the nephrologist and discovered that I would lose my right kidney, I was really distraught. I called Cliff and he met me at home at noon. Cliff, Drew, and I were sitting in the kitchen when Karen called from California to offer moral support. We'd been calmly discussing the ramifications of my medical situation, but I hadn't yet told Cliff and Drew the nephrologist's diagnosis.

As soon as I heard Karen's voice, I started to cry and sobbed, "I'm going to lose my kidney." I hope that was a rare incidence of self-pity.

KAREN

The nadir of this hellacious period was one day when I called my parents during my 15-minute break between classes. At this point, all we knew was that Mom had cancer, most likely ovarian. As soon as my mom answered the phone, she started to cry. I walked out of the campus courtyard toward the parking lot in the hope that I would find a bit of privacy. She told me that the doctors had confirmed that she had ovarian cancer, and that it had spread to one of her kidneys. I felt like someone had ripped out my heart.

My mind raced as I sat through the hour and three-quarters of my next class. Would Mom need a kidney transplant? Was I a tissue match — could I be the donor? How extensive would the surgery be, and when? Would I be able to get home for it? Above all, would she make it and could I even imagine if she didn't?

I went for a run after class, pounding through the campus loop in a new record time while my mind set running records of its own. When I got back to my room, I called home again.

Mom felt terrible that she'd told me between classes. She said that she'd actually debated whether to tell me or not, given that I was so far away and she didn't want to worry me.

Worry me?

"How can I deal with being so far away if I'm not certain that you'll tell me everything? I'm part of this family too and I need to know that you are being honest with me." I realized I was almost yelling at her, and took a deep breath before continuing.

"Mom, please promise me that you will tell me everything that happens — good and bad. If I don't know that you're doing that, I'll always assume the worst."

Even though she acquiesced and promised to tell me everything, I still felt shattered after our call. I knocked on Sarah's door, but she wasn't there. I tried to read for class, but couldn't focus on a word.

So I called Geordie, whom I'd been dating casually for all of two weeks.

"Hey, what're you up to?" I asked. He was just sitting around. "Do you want to go for a drive?"

As he drove, I talked to him for the first time about my mom's situation. It was somehow easier to talk in a moving car, looking straight ahead with a bit of distance between us. He told me that his mother had also had cancer — breast cancer, twice, over ten years ago. When he shared his regret from being away from home for both of her mastectomies, it strengthened my resolve to be home for the entire week of my mom's surgery.

VICKI

Suddenly I realized I had cancer — and a bad diagnosis at that. I began to think about all of the things I would miss because I was sure I was going to die — Karen's and Drew's weddings (although neither was engaged and Karen had just barely started dating someone new), grandchildren, retirement, time to travel and do the things I had looked forward to having time for. I'm afraid I didn't give much thought to what the rest of the family would go through without me. I had struggled with depression for years, and was finally making some progress when the greatest depressant of all — cancer — was setting me back.

I cried myself to sleep every night and woke up to more tears. I must have been very difficult for my family to deal with. I also had to tell my sister, Cyndi, about it. She was 15 years younger than me, just 39, and still considering having children. Now, as the sister of someone with ovarian cancer, she had a risk factor she hadn't counted on.

During the day, I struggled to get work done at the office with all my co-workers wanting to tell me how sorry they were and extending their best wishes. While I truly appreciated their sentiments, they took a lot of time and a great emotional toll when I was trying to meet deadlines while having medical appointments and feeling just terrible.

KAREN
Over the next few days, I spoke with professors to get time off from classes, scheduled my flights, and did several weeks of work in one. A classmate who was a doctor generously spent several hours helping me understand the information I'd heard, and I started to make sense of the CA-125 blood test results, cancer treatment options, and the future ramifications of losing a kidney. I looked for additional information on the Internet and what I found was generally dismal. No statistic I saw gave my mother

better than a one-in-three chance of surviving more than five years.

During the first weeks following Mom's diagnosis, I'd discovered that talking to some people could ease my mind, while others made everything seem even worse than it was. Even with Sarah next door, my friend Becky was my first port of call. Not only was she one of my Harvard room-mates, but like me, she'd lived in San Francisco since graduation so I'd probably spent more time with her than anyone else in the last few years. Becky had endless stamina — for sports as much as socializing — and had a matter of fact manner I found refreshing, especially now.

I flew home on the day of the Stanford vs. University of California, Berkeley football game. As I waited for Becky to pick me up, I saw cars lined up along Campus Drive, barely crawling along. I tried to call her on her cell phone to warn her to take another route, but all of the signals were taken by people coordinating tailgates and meeting places for the "Big Game" — the most important and social sports event of the season. When Becky finally got to me in her little red Subaru, we avoided Campus Drive and sped to the airport.

As we approached the departure lane at San Francisco International Airport, my nervousness of being late for my flight switched to anxiety about the trip. Becky saw me off with a strong hug and a promise that I could call whenever I wanted or needed to. I took her up on her offer and called as soon as I'd checked in for my flight — just five minutes after leaving her car. We talked until I boarded.

When I emerged from the gate at Dulles, I quickly found my parents — Mom in a jumper as she'd warned me she would be. She'd described her new look as "pregnant", and I hated admitting to myself that she was right. When we got home, she showed me her distended abdomen, swollen beyond what I could have imagined.

VICKI

My surgery was scheduled for Monday, November 22nd, 1999.

On Sunday, my dear friends Nancy and Carole came to the house with good wishes and a light blue flannel nightgown with clouds on it. They said that it was to remind me of the blue skies ahead. I have so many wonderful friends — and didn't realize how many or how wonderful until this surgery brought them together.

SURGERY
Thanksgiving Week 1999

VICKI

I'll confess that I went into surgery with little preconceived notion about what it would be like. I knew that it would take a couple of hours because of the dual surgeries involved. The first surgery would be performed by a gynecologic oncologist, and I was pleased to learn that my gynecologist would be assisting. Then a urologist would remove my kidney and the oncologist would come back to stitch me up — or rather staple me up with the most heavy-duty staples I'd ever seen. Cliff and Karen would be waiting for me to emerge from the anesthesia in the intensive care unit.

We arrived at the hospital very early as requested. After registering, I shivered in my thin hospital gown while Karen, Cliff, and I waited for the doctors to arrive.

KAREN

While we waited, Dad took one of her hands and held it in his, stroking her forearm gently with his other hand. The anesthesiologist and medical resident answered our questions as they prepared Mom for her surgery. Of course, they couldn't answer the question I was afraid to ask: would she be OK?

When they were ready to take her, Dad released her hand and softly embraced her. I leaned over to kiss her cheek and gave her shoulder a goodbye squeeze. We exchanged nervous smiles as they wheeled her away.

VICKI

I bid goodbye with a smile to Cliff and Karen and went off to a brightly-lit room. There were myriad spotlights suspended in banks from the ceiling and lots of folks dressed in operating room scrubs. That's all I remember until I "came to" in the recovery room.

KAREN

After they wheeled Mom away, Dad and I took her clothes and leg brace out to the car and went down to the hospital cafeteria for breakfast. Then, we returned to the aptly-named waiting room, where I looked up in anticipation whenever the doors opened. After about two hours, I confessed to Dad that I was nervous that we hadn't heard anything yet.

He tried to reassure me with his reply. "I'd be more concerned if the doctors had come out quickly. When Apa had his surgery for colon cancer, the doctors came out almost immediately to tell us that his cancer was so advanced that removing it would be pointless. They just closed him up and started palliative treatment."

I hadn't thought about my grandfather in a long time, since he'd died when I was only five years old. Now, I suddenly realized that Dad was only 34 when he lost his father — just eight years older than I was now. Dad always seemed ageless to me — the six foot half inch tall, fit man sitting next to me looked almost exactly the same as he had in pictures from when I was a young child. Even his short brown hair still had only the faintest hint of gray.

I thought, "Wow, he would have looked like this when he lost his dad; and now he may lose his wife."

As those thoughts came to me, my eyes stung and I tried to push them away. Dad noticed and with a gentle smile, he quietly took my hand.

After a few hours, a silver-haired man in surgical scrubs came out and introduced himself as the gynecologic oncologist. He had just performed the first part of the surgery in which his team removed Mom's ovaries, fallopian tubes, uterus and cervix, in addition to part of her colon — but not enough to require a colostomy. Mom was now in the hands of the urologist, who would be removing her right kidney. Then, the oncologist and his team would return to "staple her up".

Dad and I ate a quick lunch, and then resumed our waiting game — oscillating between attempts at reading and pacing the floor.

More than eight hours after my mom had gone into surgery, the oncologist came out again. He had deep circles under his eyes, but his kind, gentle smile remained. He deemed the surgery a success, calling the result "optimal de-bulking". This means that any cancer left in her body was less than one centimeter in diameter and optimal for treatment with chemotherapy. However, he cautioned us that her cancer was quite advanced, at Stage IIIC. This meant that it had spread substantially beyond her ovaries. Altogether, they'd taken over eight masses to be biopsied. He left us with no doubt that she still had a tough battle to wage with the cancer.

We battered him with questions that he patiently answered.

"What is the process from here?"

She would be in the intensive care unit (ICU) overnight so they could watch her. He reminded us of the extent of her surgery. Her incision went from the center of her rib cage all the way down to her pubic bone. The surgeons had literally lifted all of her abdominal organs and looked between, around, and behind them to check for tumors. With that level of physical trauma, her body would have a slow recovery. She'd be on an artificial respirator until the following morning and probably on intravenous fluids and medications for most of the week.

"When will she be able to go home?"

As soon as her body starts working again so she can eat and drink normally. This could take anywhere from four to eight days.

Thank goodness I'd planned to stay home for a week!

"Was chemotherapy absolutely necessary?"

Yes. The surgeons had taken out all the cancer they could, but some small masses remained and would certainly grow, if left untreated.

Dad and I exchanged anxious looks. Some of Mom's parting words pre-surgery were that she'd go through with the surgery, but she would NOT do chemotherapy afterward. Either the surgery would work, or it wouldn't, but that would be the end of treatment for her. She did not want to become "a cancer patient". I dreaded having her find out that her ordeal was far from over.

"Will she lose her hair?"

Unfortunately she would almost certainly lose her hair on the recommended chemotherapy regimen of Taxol and Carboplatin, but it would grow back.

A few minutes later, Dad and I went to the ICU to see her and I held back my tears as I saw how utterly weak and fragile she looked. She was unconscious, as we'd been told she would be. Her skin was ashen, a stark contrast to her short cropped, raven hair. She had tubes everywhere — small tubes in her arm and nose, electrodes checking her heart function, and a large breathing tube in her mouth. We stood next to her for a few minutes, before finally leaving to go home.

VICKI

After quite some time in recovery I heard the nurse saying that I would be "coming to" very soon. I tried to open my eyes and to talk but nothing happened. My body "came to" in lots of little stages. When I could finally open my eyes, I still couldn't move my arms or legs. They seemed glued to the bed. I'm sure that what followed for the next hours was quite standard. I didn't try to remember the details then and I don't remember them now. So much happened later that was of greater significance that the post-op details don't seem relevant to my story.

KAREN

When we arrived at the hospital the next morning, Mom was awake and her breathing tube had been removed.

After a soft kiss hello, her first words to me were, "I'm so glad you changed out of that heinous orange shirt!"

So much for my effort to dress cheerfully for her surgery, but at least her jibe was a good indication for her recovery.

I replied that I'd worn my orange shirt the day before and had changed into something else this morning.

Mom was surprised to learn that an entire day had passed — she'd been unconscious for most of it.

VICKI

I was automatically assigned to a single room. I really appreciated that — especially after the flowers began to arrive. There were so many floral arrangements that I had to ask Cliff to take them home in stages to make room for more. If there's any one common characteristic about my family, friends, and co-workers, it's that they know how to send lots of flowers and notes. Tracking and acknowledging them all was challenging.

Cliff and Karen were with me for most of my waking hours that week. Other visitors included first and foremost my dear friend Nancy. We met when Drew and her son were toddlers and she's been one of my best friends ever since. She was so thoughtful to just come to cheer me up each day, and stay no longer than my attention span could handle.

Drew and his girlfriend, my sister Cyndi, and my in-laws Carolyn and Ted were the other relatives that came at least once while I was in the hospital. I surely wasn't very attractive in my hospital gown and post-op pallor, so I hoped I wouldn't have much company, although I enjoyed every visit.

One surprise visitor was my therapist, Carter. Although she lives in Georgetown near the hospital, I was surprised and grateful that she overrode her own strict rule about seeing me outside her office. Carter had been helping me with my depression for nearly a decade and her visit really gave me a lift. My partner, Randy, and other work colleagues and friends came to see me as well. I hesitate to prepare a list of other visitors for fear of omitting someone.

When I was awake, I was easily bored unless I had visitors. Even with Cliff and Karen, there wasn't much to talk about after a while. One afternoon, I began to draft the annual Christmas letter that accompanies our card each year. We'd had quite a wonderful year with vacations and both children's graduate programs. I wanted to focus on those, but I knew the cancer and surgery needed to be included too.

I wrote the whole letter as customary, and then Karen and Drew amended the last paragraph to say that I had last been seen walking laps around the hospital's cancer ward. It's true that I had to walk as much as I could, but it was complicated by the fact that I still needed to wear the boot and use crutches and manage the IV medications that went everywhere with me. Hopefully my orthopedist won't be reading this and finding out that I wasn't very diligent about the crutches. I was at the limit of what I could bear.

KAREN

We settled into a routine that evolved through the week. Each day, I woke up to run with Dad or lift weights in the basement, and then I ran errands for my parents or did schoolwork until hospital visiting hours started at eleven o'clock. I was at the hospital with Mom most days until visiting hours ended at eight thirty at night, unless she fell asleep earlier in the evening. Dad worked at his office every morning and came to see Mom at the hospital for most of the afternoon and evening. Drew came when he could, working around his psychology classes and his internship as a counselor at a youth shelter.

Sometimes I stayed in the room when Mom had other visitors, but I often read in the waiting room to give her a break. She must have been tired of me by the end of the week.

After hospital hours, my friends kept me company by phone. When Geordie called and asked how I was, I replied with detail about Mom's surgery and her recovery.

He let me finish, and then said, "I'm really glad that your mom's doing well, but that's not what I asked. How are *you* doing?"

Geordie was the first and only person that week who asked that question with concern only for how I was holding up. I'd been keeping myself together by focusing on my family. With Geordie's concern, my exhaustion struck me and I was overwhelmed by the emotions I felt. When we got off the phone, I felt completely raw, but also relieved. There was someone looking out for me — someone I didn't have to be strong for. That night, I cried myself to sleep.

Despite her walks around the ward, Mom's body was still out of commission from the surgery. Each day we hoped that she'd finally be able to pass gas — and therefore go home from the hospital. Our family is not one that generally discusses bodily functions, so at first it was odd to talk about any aspect of the excretory system. Soon, however, our inhibitions were behind us and we were like cheerleaders when she'd go to her bathroom to try. Finally, on Saturday, her body finally cooperated and everyone in the room cheered when she had a little fart and went to the bathroom. She came home the next morning.

VICKI

Shortly after I came home on Sunday, Karen had to return to California and her classes. It was probably just as well for me because I really needed to rest. I appreciated more than she will ever know the sacrifice of class time and experiences with friends that she made in order to spend the entire week with me.

CONVALESCENCE
December 1999

VICKI

While I was at the hospital, Cliff had made two major changes to the house. First, he gave my old treadmill to a friend and bought me a new super-duper one. The treadmill had been my exercise mainstay for several years and we had talked about upgrading to one that would have automatic incline adjustment, et cetera. Yet, that part of my recovery seemed far away; at this point I didn't even want to think about getting on it. In fact, I was a little resentful that he'd spent the time while I was in the hospital buying it without consulting me.

The other change was to rent a hospital bed for my comfort. Cliff knew it would be difficult for me to get myself up when he was at work because my incision was still so raw and painful. So he rigged a long rope (actually a line left over from our sailing days) so that I could pull up on it rather than rely on my stomach muscles. I had gained so much weight from fluid retention in the hospital that I came home weighing in at over 180 pounds! In the first four days home I lost 40 pounds — all fluid I'm sure — so I spent lots of time pulling myself up and getting out of bed for the bathroom. This certainly wasn't much fun, but I didn't expect it to be.

Cliff came with me to my first post-op visit with the oncologist. First, a nurse removed the staples from my incision — with a staple remover, of course. My scar extended from my boobs to my belly button and beyond.

Before my surgery, I had insisted that I would not do chemo. But the doctor told us that my cancer had metastasized; it was a systemic disease that I had to fight systemically with chemotherapy. He recommended that I begin with the standard preferred first-line treatment for ovarian cancer — a combination of Carboplatin and Taxol.

The oncology nurse weighed and measured me for the chemo dosage. How could I possibly be only 5'5" when I'd been 5'7" for my entire adult life? I not only had cancer; I was shorter as well!

The nurse spent a lot of time explaining the chemotherapy process and expectations to us.

I would lose my hair. I would experience some nausea, but there were wonderful drugs to minimize that. I would be tired. But I could certainly return to work if I wanted to as long as I paced myself — no easy task in public accounting.

She recommended several wig shops in the area. I also asked my hair stylist, Eli, and went to one that had been mentioned by both. I wasn't psychologically ready to go yet, but I had heard that it's best to get a wig before the hair falls out so the styling could be as similar as possible to my own hairdo. I chose a wig called the Jackie and waited to have it fitted. The basic framework of the wig would be altered to fit my scalp, and I would return the following week to have it styled.

Just like all of this medical stuff, it takes more than one visit to accomplish anything. Drew was kind enough to drive me to both wig appointments because I still wasn't driving myself.

Drew's master's program included an internship as counselor at a nearby teen shelter. He worked twenty hours a week at the internship as well as keeping up his classes, homework, and papers, not to mention caring for Simba, his energetic Rhodesian Ridgeback puppy. Even with his busy schedule, he continued to be my chauffeur until I could drive again and he did lots of the errands to help Cliff.

KAREN

After Thanksgiving, I felt guilty for leaving my family to go back to school, but also relieved. I returned to a flood of term papers, group projects, and exams, which absorbed most of my time. I still spoke to and emailed my parents and Drew nearly every day.

With time, I started to compartmentalize more — to focus on schoolwork, friends, and Geordie without always living through the lens of Mom's health. Unlike me, my brother wasn't able to extricate himself. He was living at home and was there whenever Mom needed something. I knew about her ups and downs — and in those days there were many more downs than ups — from our calls and emails, but could briefly escape when I hung up my phone or shut down my computer. He couldn't.

VICKI

One of the kindest and most appreciated gestures while I was convalescing at home happened mid-week. Nancy and her husband called to say they were bringing over some carryout dinner. No prep work. No dishes. No mess. They came, we enjoyed a wonderful meal and conversation, and they left. I was tired, but had eaten dinner with friends. How I had missed that!

Another welcome relief from my cancer recovery came the second Saturday in December. A year earlier, Nancy had invited a few friends to join her on the second Saturday of every month for a "ladies-only" breakfast at a restaurant. I already knew two of the women and would get to know the others quite well over time: Carole, Claire, Jean, and Willie. That first December, we splurged and had breakfast at the Ritz Carlton; we decided that the Ritz Carlton would become our annual December destination.

Before my surgery, I told the group that I wouldn't see them at the Ritz this December. I had bragged to them just the month before that my family doesn't get cancer (we all die of heart attacks). A month later, I had to admit to them that I was breaking ground as first in my family to be diagnosed with ovarian cancer.

My friends rallied as usual and decided to bring breakfast to my home instead. The ladies brought food and Cliff made coffee and orange juice. It was such a thoughtful event and was definitely a very special part of Christmas for me that year. I was really excited to show off my new thinner post-surgery figure and hadn't yet started to lose my hair. Life was good. Funny, how my criteria for the "good life" had changed almost overnight. Now a good life meant no pain, lots of sleep, and a head full of hair.

A week later, I started chemotherapy. Anyone who saw the kit of distractions I took to the first chemo would certainly be amused. I didn't normally pack so much for a week at the beach! I had a tape recorder with earphones to listen to music, a couple of novels, a journal, crossword puzzles, needlepoint, and a large lunch.

While several people had offered to drive me to chemo and stay with me, it really wasn't necessary. Drew drove me over and picked me up at the end of the day. The nurses were right there with me and Drew was available to come over if an emergency occurred or if I needed to come home early. Besides, I wasn't sure how this would go for me and I didn't want to have friends or family in attendance. It really bothered me that I was now known as the cancer patient, when I had previously been known as just the mother or wife or accountant or friend. Those titles suited me much better.

Once the treatment started, I tried reading but couldn't get into either book. Needlepoint was too difficult with the IV in my wrist. But I could do the crossword puzzles with no difficulty. I also tried writing in the journal that Karen's friend Anne-Marie had given me to chronicle my post-op experiences. But the journal was lovely, with recycled pages decorated with what looked like rose petals. How could I possibly write about anything as gruesome as this experience in such a lovely book? True to form, I described what I was wearing and listed the items I'd brought for distractions. Just nothing medical or personal.

After surgery, my CA-125 had plummeted from 1200 to 65. I felt I was almost home free. Now we just needed to get rid of the microscopic cells that remained after the surgery. My next CA-125 wouldn't be done for another two weeks and I could hardly wait for it.

After all the chemo was finished, the nurse gave me instructions and good wishes for recovering at home. I was relieved that the nausea wasn't nearly as bad as I had expected from reading memoirs of cancer patients. Then, about a week after the first chemo treatment I developed an angry, red rash all over my body. The oncologist insisted that the rash wasn't related to the chemotherapy, but I couldn't think what else would have caused it. I went to see our family's dermatologist, who agreed with me that the rash was probably caused by the Taxol. He recommended regular doses of Benadryl and oatmeal baths. At first the baths repulsed me, but I was soon looking forward to them because they were so soothing to my inflamed skin.

KAREN

After my fall term exams, I joined some friends in Lake Tahoe for a few days in the mountains before going back to Virginia. I decided to try snowboarding for the first time, and almost immediately regretted my choice. By the first run of my lesson — if you could call my snail's pace a run — I had already fallen on my bum so many times that I felt the bruises forming. I started the second run frustrated and determined to do better. I had finally started to pick up a little speed when I lost control. I instinctively put out my left arm to break my fall. As I struck the snow, I heard a snap, and a sharp pain exploded in my wrist.

A few hours later, I was in the local hospital looking at an x-ray that confirmed the break in my forearm. Drew answered the phone when I called my family.

"Hey Ruf, is Dad there?" Ruf was my nickname for Drew since we were young — I'd morphed Drew into Drewfer, then Rufer, and finally Ruf.

"No."

"Is Mom there?"

"She's taking a nap." His impatient tone made it clear that I'd interrupted him.

"Can you help me then? I just broke my wrist snowboarding and I need you to change my airline ticket to come home earlier."

"I'm in the middle of writing a paper. Do you need me to call right now?"

"Ruf, are you kidding me? I just broke my wrist! It hurts and I want to get on an earlier flight. My cell phone doesn't work here and I can't exactly use the hospital phone to wait on hold with the airline." As my voice rose, I could sense the nurses giving me space.

"Don't yell at me! Hold on, I'll get Mom."

"No! Don't wake her up!" But he'd already gone to get her.

Mom sounded groggy when she got on the phone but, as always, she took care of everything. When I called back from the ski house a few hours later, she'd already changed my flight and paid the change fee.

Under normal circumstances, a broken arm merits loads of sympathy. Mine generated ironic laughter. Given Dad's slashed thumb and broken wrist that fall, and Mom's stress fracture and cancer, another broken wrist wasn't even noteworthy. It was just a nuisance that impeded my ability to help out at home.

Just as Mom had warned me before Thanksgiving that she'd be in a jumper, this time she'd reminded me that she'd be without hair. She also doubted that she'd have enough energy to come to the airport with Dad to meet me. As the plane touched down, I wondered if this would be the first time her warning came true. For my entire life, BOTH of my parents had ALWAYS met me at the airport gate, unless they had an absolutely necessary conflict. Was she so sick that her need to rest at home counted as an urgent conflict?

I was relieved to see them both in the waiting area, Dad waving vigorously while Mom stood beside him smiling. She looked tiny, engulfed in her long, navy blue wool coat with a hat on her head. When I hugged her, she felt so much smaller — and weaker — than any other time I remembered. I worried that she was just wasting away.

VICKI

The highlight of Christmas that year was having Karen home again. Unfortunately she had joined the ranks of the injured and infirm. Had one of us broken a mirror we didn't know about? Drew was currently the only Greve left unscathed.

Christmas was on Saturday that year, just eight days after my chemo, and I still had a residual, very itchy, rash. As was customary, we went to Christmas Eve services followed by dinner out with Cliff's sister Carolyn and her family. Throughout dinner, I tried to unobtrusively scratch my back by moving gently against the back of the seat. I was so uncomfortable, but determined not to make my discomfort an issue.

KAREN

This visit home was different, as Mom's cancer was an omnipresent reminder that things had changed. I felt like an interloper, intruding on the routine that my family had in place. I wanted to help, but was limited in how much I could do because of my arm. Not only was it broken, but because of the position of the break, my cast went from three inches below my armpit to my hand, bending at the elbow. At least I'd persuaded the doctor to make the angle a natural one for running. I'd just started training for the Napa Marathon in March, and knew I'd go crazy if I couldn't run off my stress.

My poor brother had his own stress that Christmas. When I called from the hospital in Tahoe, he'd been helping my parents through injuries and ailments for several months, while studying and working full-time. When I started to see how harried he was, I understood his frustration on the phone. I had needed his help, but he was probably in even greater need than I was — not to have to help anyone. On top of everything else, he and his girlfriend were breaking up after five years together.

We all really wanted to have a "normal" Christmas, despite everything. Part of a normal Christmas for our family meant baking the same seven types of Christmas cookies that Dad's family has made for generations: Lebkuchen, chocolate stars, "S" cookies, brown sugar cookies, Russian tea cakes, rocks, and Springerle. Baking was a group effort this year, with Mom instructing from the sofa between naps, while Dad and I mixed and baked, and Drew took study breaks to sample our progress.

In addition to cookies, another part of a "normal" Greve Christmas is an obscene abundance of gifts under the tree. But even unwrapping presents on Christmas morning, cancer made its presence felt. Among her other gifts, Mom must have gotten ten hats and scarves under the tree for her newly shaved head. Two of them were from me: a gorgeous grey faux-fur for dress up; the other was a floppy green corduroy for gardening and casual wear.

So, much as we tried to have a "normal" Christmas, it was anything but. After a whirlwind three-week visit, I was soon on a flight back to California.

TEAL RIBBON
January – March 2000

VICKI

On New Year's Eve, we went to a dinner party at Nancy's home. I wore a size 10 velvet dress that I hadn't been able to wear in years and was delighted to be so thin, especially since I had already lost my hair.

About two weeks after chemo, my hair had started to fall out whenever I touched it, combed it, or showered and shampooed. At the end of a shower, it completely covered the drain. The thinning occurred in the front and sides at first, causing my face to look so much older. Soon, there was very little left. One Saturday, I went to my regular hair stylist, Eli, after the salon closed and the other customers and staff had left. He had recently lost his mother to a lengthy battle with cancer and was very sensitive to the special needs of cancer patients. In the privacy of the back room, he shaved my head down to stubble. What a shock! Actually, it felt and looked much better to be shaved than to have scraggly gray hair. I was relieved that my head was finally neat and manageable again.

At the infusion center, I discovered two sources for hats and scarves designed especially for cancer patients. I bought way too many of them; my collection is impressive. At first I wore hats almost exclusively because I thought the wig was heinous — although it was really quite nice. But the hats aged me because they were so severe. They had looked lovely in the catalogs when modeled by women with eyebrows and eyelashes. On my hairless face, they just looked drab. One special hat I bought was a nightcap. On winter nights, my head was quite cold without any hair. I bought the nightcap in both pink and blue and loved it. I developed a new appreciation for bald people. How do they cope — and without complaining?

KAREN

To add insult to injury, my mother's natural hair was striking. She called it her best feature, but I think it's one of many. For my entire life, she'd worn the same close-cut salt and pepper hairstyle. The only difference over the years was how the salt had gradually started to dominate the pepper. I couldn't imagine her in the bland, grey-brown wig she'd bought as a temporary replacement.

I spent the Millennium New Year in a cabin in Lake Tahoe, with ten friends including Geordie and Becky. It was a relaxed holiday with days spent outdoors and evenings lounging in front of a roaring fire in our cozy cabin.

While my friends skied, I started training for my fifth marathon, the Napa Valley Marathon in March. On New Year's Eve Day, I set out on a twelve mile run along the mountain highway. As I ran along the icy terrain, I focused on two things: not falling on my broken arm and a conversation with Mom the week before.

We'd been having an earnest conversation about how she was and what I could do to make things easier for her. She said that there wasn't anything — it just helped to know that I loved her and was just a phone call or email away. At least, that was how she felt most of the time. She admitted that sometimes she wished she could ask me to move back home to be with her.

I quickly reassured her that I was always available by phone except when I was in a class, and that I would come home for the weekend as often as she wanted me to. I didn't offer to leave school and she didn't mention it again.

Part of me felt that I should quit my MBA and go home, but most of my heart and mind rebelled against the thought. I'd spent the last eight years of my life working toward where I was right now and hoped my Stanford MBA would open amazing career opportunities to me. Then, there was Geordie. I had started falling in love with him before Christmas and seeing him again over the New Year reinforced my feelings. As much as I realized that we were far from making a long-term commitment, I thought that it was very possible that he was "the one" for me. But, I didn't think we were ready to build our relationship from across the continent.

Geordie's mother, Vivian, came to Palo Alto for a visit that winter and shared her own experience with breast cancer. Vivian insisted that she wouldn't have wanted Geordie to stop his life experiences to be there for her radiation treatments and was certain that Mom felt the same way.

As she said, somewhat defiantly, "What would Geordie have done at home — chauffeur me to appointments? I could drive myself, thank you very much."

Geordie always spoke with pride about his parents, and described his mom as a brilliant woman whose determination took her beyond her poor, rural Ontario village to a self-financed honors degree from Queen's, one of Canada's top universities, where she met his dad. I could see why he was proud of her; his mom's perseverance reminded me of my own mother's experience as one of the first from her small town to graduate from college.

Vivian's advice resonated with me: what would I do at home? I couldn't start in a professional position with the caveat that I'd need frequent breaks during the work week for doctor's appointments with my mother. Going home without a job seemed absurd — after all, Mom intended to go back to work, so chauffeuring her to appointments wouldn't constitute a full-time commitment.

This issue continued to haunt me through the remainder of my MBA. Fortunately, Mom never again raised the idea of my moving back home. Her selflessness offset my selfishness almost perfectly.

VICKI

My second week back at work, I traveled with my colleagues to a training seminar in Dallas, Texas. With my wig. With my fatigue. With my nausea and constipation, because I had had chemo the Wednesday before I left. I had handled lots of challenges in the past, so surely I could handle this as well. It was so wonderful to see everyone and show them that I had survived and was doing well. I was so happy to see one colleague that I shocked her with a huge bear hug — and almost lost my wig in the process. But, the training schedule was arduous for me. After eight hours of meetings, the group all went out for dinner together each night and I didn't want to miss anything.

January is typically slow for our practice. By slow, I mean 40 hours a week instead of 60 or 70. Plus, I had to contend with chemo treatments and blood tests. I was exhausted, sleeping all day most weekends and going to bed right after dinner during the week. This wasn't a dream life, but I was determined to keep my job while recovering from cancer. I hoped this recovery period would be short.

Months before my diagnosis, Cliff and Drew had scheduled a duck hunting trip for the weekend of the Martin Luther King, Jr. holiday in January. They offered to cancel their plans to stay home with me, but instead Karen graciously agreed to come home so I wouldn't be alone for the weekend. We had a very low-key visit, and it was wonderful to spend time with just the two of us. In character, I was well enough to take Karen to dinner at our favorite French restaurant.

KAREN

In February, Drew literally "broke" his distinction as the only uninjured Greve when he fractured several bones in his foot playing basketball. Like my arm, it was almost comic . . . almost. The family tally now included Dad's slashed left thumb and broken right wrist, my broken left wrist, Drew's broken foot and Mom's stress fracture and cancer. Not that cancer equates to a broken bone — by relative hardship, Mom was still leagues ahead of the rest of us.

I felt as though I'd gotten off easily, relative to the rest of my family. My arm was healing well and I was on track for a personal best marathon time in Napa. When my cast was removed in early February, my run times got even better as I lost a couple of pounds on the left side of my body!

Then, two weeks before the race, I felt a pain in my left groin area. It worsened every day and on my final training run before my Sunday race, it was excruciating. I'd run for less than two minutes when I stopped, turned, and walked slowly back to the dorm. I couldn't hold back my tears when I called Geordie. I really wanted to do this race. I felt like I needed it to maintain my identity as an athlete.

As an athlete himself, Geordie understood my desire to race through the pain, but also the absurdity of doing so. He crafted the perfect argument to convince me not to run — reminding me that I'd run marathons before and had nothing to prove — and was no longer in any condition to achieve a personal best time. I knew he was right, yet I didn't believe it until a CT scan confirmed that I had a stress fracture in my left femur (thigh bone). It would be months before I was able to run again and my wrist was still too weak to lift weights or even to swim. I'd lost my exercise outlet during a time when I really needed it for my emotional stability.

Both of my parents met me at the airport when I flew back for my spring break. On my last two trips home, Mom had warned me about her appearance. She hadn't done so this time and I was shocked at how much older she looked. Her eyebrows and eyelashes had fallen out since Christmas, aging her by more than ten years. At least she was more comfortable with her hairless state. She scarcely ever wore her wig or hats at home, preferring to be comfortable *au naturel*. Within a few days, I was used to her new look. The good news was that it seemed like it would be temporary.

At least, Mom's CA-125 tests indicated that her chemo-therapy was winning the war against cancer. Her test results had gone from 1200 to 65 after the surgery, then to 33 after the first month of chemo and then to 15 and most recently 14. All three most recent results were below the magic threshold of 35. The doctor reminded us that this did not mean that she was healed, and she needed to finish the full regimen of Carboplatin and Taxol through April, but all indications were that she was on the road to remission.

It was obvious that her work schedule and treatment regimen were taking their toll, yet she seldom complained. Actually, when she did complain, it was often that she felt like we didn't adequately understand how sick she was because she didn't complain about it. She was right. She coped with such grace that sometimes we forgot that she usually didn't feel well, that her food tasted terrible, that she had numbness in her hands and feet, and that she was always tired.

VICKI
One of the first chemotherapy side effects I noticed was neuropathy, tingling and loss of feeling in my fingertips and toes. Dressing in blouses with buttons and French cuffs was proving to be difficult. Another side effect of my chemo was that it was very hard on my red and white blood cells, which is why I was so very tired. By February, they were both so low that I had to take shots of a drug called Procrit. There was no way I would be able to stick myself with a needle, so Cliff agreed to give me the needed shots, just as he had given me allergy shots for years before.

KAREN

One of Mom's chemo nurses gave her two "teal ribbon" pins, fashioned after the pink ribbons worn in support of finding a cure for breast cancer. Mom gave one of them to me and I wore it every day, including the day of Dad's cataract surgery, for which I was his chauffeur.

His surgery was a complete success and he was amazed at how much clearer and brighter the world looked without cataracts. For me, the world had started to look brighter before he even left the waiting room for his surgery.

As we waited for him to be called back, I noticed that the nurse was wearing a pin similar to the one Mom had given me. I asked her if it was for ovarian cancer and surprise registered on her face that I'd recognized it.

The nurse was an eleven-year survivor of Stage IIIB ovarian cancer, almost the same stage as Mom! She was a stunning woman about Mom's age, with close cropped salt and pepper hair similar in style to my mother's before chemo. She was still on chemotherapy, and had been almost continuously since her diagnosis. Yet, she was vibrant and full of energy. She worked full-time and participated in all local walks for the cure. I dreaded the thought that Mom could be on cancer treatments for the next decade, but preferred that to losing her prematurely. Dad's nurse helped me to believe that Mom could, and would, survive this disease.

VICKI

I had my last treatment of Carboplatin and Taxol in April. I was just delighted to be rid of cancer forever. I was sure I had beaten the odds.

REMISSION
April – October 2000

VICKI

My sister Cyndi is fifteen years younger than I am and we had been quite close for most of her life. So, I was disappointed that she didn't take a greater interest in me and my cancer once I was diagnosed. She did stop by to see me for a short visit in the hospital, but she didn't come to the house until I'd been home for a couple of weeks.

Then one day, she brought me a small pillow that said "It's good to be queen." I just chuckled at it. Another day, she stopped on the way home from work and brought some English toasting bread she had made. Just small gestures, but greatly appreciated. I suspect that she must have had almost as great a shock as I did when I was diagnosed. I had always been the strong older sister and had helped to take care of her when she was a young girl. Now I was sick, and who knew if I would overcome this malady. Little did I know that her attention to me and my recovery was about to kick into overdrive.

In January 2000, Cyndi called to ask if I would be interested in attending the retreat in April that her quilters' guild was planning. The retreat would require that I take off from work on Friday, returning home by mid-afternoon on Sunday. Although my energy was really not at top level, I agreed to go. I was actually looking forward to it because I had loved to sew all my life and hadn't done any meaningful sewing since making prom and cotillion dresses for Karen when she was in high school. I wasn't even sure my sewing machine would still work. I'd bought it when Karen was born and had really used it hard over the years. This one had replaced my first machine, on which I'd made my gown and Cyndi's flower girl dress for my wedding, over thirty years ago.

Could I survive three days at the Four-H Center with 64 other women just eating, sleeping, talking, and most of all, sewing?

The theme of the retreat was UFOs (Un-Finished Projects) so I took the quilt I had started for Karen when she was in the eighth grade. I actually won a prize at the retreat for the oldest unfinished project! I took my wig, but hid under my hats for most of the weekend. The other women were friendly and considerate, but I was painfully aware that they had never met me as just a 54 year-old. They met me as Cyndi's elderly-looking sister, the cancer patient. I was generally the first to go to bed at night, but managed to get up with the others for breakfast and stick it out for the whole day. In all, it was a wonderful experience and I looked forward to future weekends of sewing with such committed quilters.

I had no idea then that Cyndi and I would soon become inseparable and that quilting and cancer would be the common bonds between us.

KAREN

Mom and Dad planned their first trip out to see me at Stanford, scheduled to coincide with the MBA program's 75th Anniversary Gala in May. I eagerly anticipated their visit and their first time meeting Geordie. They arrived on Friday and we went to dinner that evening at a chic, upscale Creole restaurant.

As soon as we sat down, Mom and I started to catch up while Dad and Geordie got to know each other as men do — by talking about sports. After a few minutes Mom stopped talking and gestured to the guys.

Their conversation was even more animated than our own — and not about sports. They were talking about their intellectual interests as an engineer (Dad) and astrophysics major (Geordie), discussing Geordie's undergraduate thesis and Dad's career. I can safely say that Geordie is my only boyfriend who ever showed the least comprehension of, much less interest in, Dad's field of photogrammetry and remote sensing. I had never really understood it myself — until Geordie explained it to me later.

Dad and Geordie seemed oblivious that they were now the subject of our conversation. Mom whispered to me that they reminded her of Dad with her father, sharing their love of photography. In my entire life, I had never seen Dad more engaged in any conversation. Mom and I spent most of the rest of the evening listening to our guys talking and enjoying their interaction. We'd been seated at seven o'clock and lingered at our table until well past ten, when jet lag finally caught up with my parents.

Geordie had to leave the next morning for a friend's bachelor party in Las Vegas, leaving me to spend the weekend with my parents. Dad told me — unsolicited, and in an excited voice — that he thought Geordie was a "neat guy, with a brilliant mind." Mom spent much of the weekend talking about how special Geordie seemed to her. She commented that I was absolutely glowing — and I felt like I was. I was in love and felt reassured that my parents not only approved of, but genuinely liked Geordie.

Saturday night we went to the gala at Stanford; it was a lavish affair. The four-course meal was served at over a hundred tables, each adorned with an opulent arrangement of roses. My parents and I were seated at a table with some of my classmates, all of whom knew what Mom had endured over the past six months. It felt like a celebration dinner — the triumphant joining of my worlds.

VICKI

For the black-tie event, I wore my old standby black evening pant suit. And, of course, my wig. The weather was uncharacteristically hot and poor Cliff was stuck in his tuxedo jacket, just like all the other men. At the dinner, we met quite a few of Karen's new friends, who were just lovely and poised, making them wonderful company for the evening.

I was much less so. Although I was able to remove my jacket, I had no choice about my wig. It was uncomfortable and hot, causing perspiration to gather non-stop on my face. I was sure I wasn't a very pretty sight, but it wasn't until I saw the pictures that I realized just how awful I looked. In my frequent blotting of the perspiration on my face, I had completely removed my painted-on eyebrows. I looked more like a mannequin with her wig askew than like a woman who actually belonged at my table. Karen and her friends were so gracious that we had a wonderful time in spite of my appearance and the heat.

KAREN

A month later, Geordie flew to New York to start his summer internship with Goldman Sachs. My own internship didn't start for another week, so I headed back east for my five year Harvard College reunion and a visit with my parents. This visit was my fifth in the eight months since Mom's diagnosis — and was completely different from the others.

Mom was a different person than she'd been the previous spring, or even in Palo Alto in May. She was back to her natural, but still very short and now much curlier, hairstyle and was free of cancer treatments. She was working hard at the office, but wasn't burdened by weekly doctor's appointments. Life felt almost back to normal. Even so, looking at my parents, I realized that they had both aged incredibly over the past year. Dad, especially, had a haggard look and predominantly gray hair that I didn't remember from just a year earlier.

A few days into my visit, I took a day trip down to Virginia farm country. Drew was working on a farm that summer for one of Dad's former colleagues. He raved about the open space for his dog, Simba, to run around in, and the kind country folk he worked with. He boarded at the farmhouse and literally worked from sunrise to well past sunset, doing hard manual labor. When I spoke with Drew on the phone, he sounded like a kid who got to play with his favorite toy every day. I was anxious to see him in his element.

After Drew engulfed me in a huge feet-off-the-ground bear hug, he admonished me for wearing shorts and sandals. It was well over 90 degrees outside and stickily humid! Clearly, I'd missed Farming 101 and didn't adequately realize the dangers of having bare legs in fields with tall grasses. As he warned me about chiggers and other vermin, I was really wondering what he loved about this place.

Then, I saw it first-hand. He gave me a tour of the restored farm house, and showed me the outbuildings where the equipment was stored — tractors with attachments that were much larger than I'd imagined they would be. His eyes were shining and he was talking so fast about so many aspects of farming that he kept interrupting himself. This was my brother at his best.

For the rest of the summer I worked at the San Francisco office of Bain & Company, a strategic management consulting firm. I was captivated by my colleagues and strategy work and decided that I wanted to work for Bain after graduation, but unfortunately not in San Francisco. I only visited my parents once that summer: I flew in on the red eye Friday night and flew back first thing Monday to return straight to work, exhausted. Plus, the time difference combined with my job constraints made it difficult to call my parents.

All indications were that Mom's cancer was under control. But it had changed me. Even though I wasn't willing to leave school and stay home, I also wasn't willing to have long periods pass without seeing or talking to my parents. Time with them seemed more precious than it had just a year earlier.

Another factor pulling me east was Geordie's job. He was excited about working for Goldman Sachs and his chosen career trading fixed income derivatives was available in only three cities: New York, London and Tokyo. New York fit my close to home criteria — being in the same time zone and only a three-hour train ride from Arlington.

I had missed Geordie after being apart for the entire summer. He wasn't much of a phone talker, and I wasn't much for going without talking, so long distance had not been an easy experience. At one point during the summer, I'd even wondered if we'd still be together at the other end of it. Happily we were, and when we were finally back together, I remembered why. I loved laughing with him. I loved the way he ran his hands through my hair as we talked. I loved it when he picked me up as though I were as light as a feather and playfully tossed me around the room. I loved sleeping in, and then waking up together. Yes, I was still in love, and wonder of all wonders, so was he.

A few days after arriving back at school that fall, I flew back east to meet the partners in Bain's New York office and make my case for a transfer.

I didn't want to make an issue of Mom's cancer, especially when she seemed to be getting better. But in the meeting, it was apparent that my "I want to move to New York to be with my boyfriend" argument wasn't helping my case for a transfer. I took a breath and offered the more urgent reason for me to move to New York: my mother had advanced stage ovarian cancer and it was important for me to be close enough to see her on weekends. As I heard my voice waver, I was frustrated at my lack of composure in a business setting. The partner seemed to sense my unease and was sympathetic, but professional.

After four agonizing weeks back at school, I found out that my transfer had gone through. In the end, my partner and manager in San Francisco had given strong endorsements and insisted that the firm permit my transfer. I was told in no uncertain terms that it was this, more than any of my personal reasons, which facilitated my transfer. I was relieved and grateful.

CHEMOTHERAPY
October 2000 – February 2001

VICKI

I don't believe that any of the MRIs done between April and October 2000 showed any additional growths. However, my CA-125 had begun to elevate again. By October it was up to 116. I could hardly believe that the cancer hadn't been cured in the spring! Wasn't my CA-125 down to 14 in March?

KAREN

For our second year of business school, my roommate, Sarah, had moved back to San Francisco, an hour from Stanford. I moved into a house near campus with my friends Katie and Lauren. It was a typical Silicon Valley home: low slung stucco, with three small bedrooms on its single floor. It was ample for three women, but became very cozy for five when Geordie and Katie's fiancé, John, were over. Fortunately for all of our sanity, our varied class schedules meant that we were seldom all home at the same time.

One evening in early October, Geordie and I had the house to ourselves. Such a treat! I snuggled up to him on the sofa while we watched football. Between classes, exercise, study groups and social outings, it seemed like we were seldom alone together. I felt warm and secure lying against him and was about to doze off when the phone rang. I was debating whether to answer it, when Geordie fished it out from under a cushion and handed it to me.

"Hi, am I interrupting anything?" It was Mom. For a second, I was tempted to say yes. She would understand if I explained that it was a rare moment alone for Geordie and me.

"No, of course not. We're just watching football. What's up?"

"I just got back from the oncologist's." Her tone gave away immediately that it hadn't been a good visit. She'd had four clear months, and with each one, I became more convinced that she'd licked her cancer. I guiltily realized that I'd forgotten about this appointment, figuring that it would be routine like the others recently.

Clearly, I was wrong. I frantically motioned for Geordie to turn the volume down until there was no sound coming from the television. He did it while I was still gesturing. His eyes caught mine and sent me strength.

"I'm glad Geordie's there with you. I don't have good news." Her cancer was back. The doctor didn't know how extensively yet, but he wanted to do a surgical procedure called a laparoscopy to check things out and remove the cancer he found.

"When's the surgery? I'll arrange my flights." At this, Geordie turned off the television and wrapped his arms tighter around me. I felt like I was suffocating and shrugged him away, getting up to walk down the hall and into my bedroom and grab a pen and notepad off my desk.

"It will probably be this week, but there's no reason for you to come back for it. It's an outpatient procedure. Your dad can go with me, or if he's busy, then Cyndi will."

"Mom, I'm not worried about who will drive you. I want to be there for you." I did; it was true. At the same time, I was in my busiest quarter yet at Stanford, with all classes deriving a significant portion of the grade from attendance and participation. I wasn't just worried that I would get a bad mark: in two of my classes, missed attendance meant failing.

Mom may have sensed my hesitation. "You need to be there at school with Geordie. Why don't you save your next visit for a time when I can enjoy being with you? I'll tell you the surgery details when I know them, but only if you promise not to come home for it."

"Are you sure?" I couldn't believe I was really asking this. I started over. "We'll see. Why don't you call me tomorrow when you hear from the doctor?"

"I will. For now, don't worry. I've survived surgery and chemo. I'll get through this too, and then we'll be scot-free."

"I'll try not to. I love you Mom."

"Oh, Karen, I love you so much. We'll talk again tomorrow."

As soon as I hung up the phone, the floodgates that I'd struggled to keep closed during our call came roaring open. I wandered back to the living room, where Geordie leapt to his feet — looking concerned.

I literally collapsed into his arms. I cried without restraint, hanging on to Geordie while he held me and stroked my hair. If he'd moved, I would have fallen to the floor. Gently, he half-carried me to the sofa and sat down with me in his lap. He never stopped stroking my hair.

"It's back. She's still sick. It didn't go away. She's having surgery in a week. She doesn't want me to come home for it. What if she doesn't make it? Why won't it go away? Why can't they just cut it out and make it go away?"

I reached for a Kleenex and blew forcefully, just hoping to be able to breathe again. As minutes passed, Geordie kept holding me, massaging my head as he ran his fingers through my hair. It felt like he was transferring his strength to my body as I cried and cried.

I suddenly realized that Mom's battle wasn't going to be a short one. Before the first surgery, I thought it would be quick — in either direction. Then, during chemotherapy, life got back into a sort of rhythm as the CA-125 numbers came down quickly and stayed down. Of course, it might come back. Cancer often did. But, even if it came back, I thought we'd have a reprieve for a few years in the meantime.

We'd had our reprieve and it lasted from April through September — six months.

Mom's surgery on October 16th "went well". It was an outpatient operation in which the oncologist removed several small spots of cancer. As Mom had suggested, I went home a week later for the Columbus Day long weekend. I wanted to see my parents, but this visit had another reason for it too. Drew was in love and I was going home to meet his girlfriend.

VICKI
One very special aspect of our family that summer was that Drew met Lynda Smith, a professional singer who lived in Mathews, VA, about an hour away from Holyoke Farm,

where Drew was working. When Drew heard Lynda sing at her family's theater, it was love at first sight. They met the following Wednesday when he persuaded her to have dinner with him.

We didn't hear much about Lynda until later in September. Drew called to say that he'd met someone very special and thought he might bring her up to meet us. We were delighted to hear about her, and even more delighted to actually meet her. She was, and is, a very special lady.

KAREN

By the time I met Lynda, it was clear that Drew had found the woman he wanted to marry and it was just a matter of timing. I loved Drew and I was happy that he was happy. But a part of me resented meeting Lynda when it was already a foregone conclusion that she would one day become my sister-in-law.

Fortunately, she is simply amazing and my petty resentment soon washed away. Lynda is like sunshine entering a room — and her long, blond mane of hair is only part of it. Vivacious is the best word I could think of to describe her, with her warm, Southern Virginia voice and easy laugh. She eventually won me over completely, but it didn't happen that weekend.

VICKI

After the laparoscopy, the oncologist said he had removed all the cancer he could see. I was impatient, but he admonished me to "hang in there" while I healed enough to start chemotherapy again. Once I was ready, he recommended Topotecan, a second-line chemotherapy that I resisted for several reasons.

First and foremost, I dreaded losing my hair again. I have felt from the beginning of this insidious illness that I could function normally and be perceived as having normal health as long as I had hair. Although I wasn't nuts about my wig, it was the facial hair I missed the most. Without hair, I would again have to brush on fresh eyebrows every morning using eye pencil, hoping they didn't smudge during the day.

I also dreaded the treatment schedule: each cycle would require chemotherapy every morning for a week straight. I found myself bringing home more and more work, getting up earlier during chemo week so I could review some tax returns before my treatments. I had 30 days of combined vacation and medical leave per year, and I was quickly using all of my time for medical appointments. Would I ever be able to take an actual vacation?

Plus, my veins couldn't sustain the frequency of this chemo regimen. After my first week on Topotecan, I went to the hospital to have a medi-port installed. It was a flat, hard contraption the size of a quarter that the doctors implanted beneath the skin on my chest to administer the chemicals directly into my vena cava. It was installed on the right side of my chest, plenty low enough for any blouse I'd have courage to wear, and high enough that my bras wouldn't bother it. To my surprise, the medi-port became one of my most positive cancer experiences, with its ease and convenience.

Somehow, I was getting used to my body being a vehicle for both cancer and its cure. My developing attitude was that I didn't care what procedures I endured, as long as they would help me get well.

Of course, fatigue continued to plague me. I began going to bed earlier and earlier. I cut out all unnecessary trips and errands, as Cliff quickly assumed responsibility for them. I just hated having that happen. He had been inconvenienced enough for a lifetime already. Now he was cooking all the meals as well as buying the groceries for them, going to the dry cleaner, drugstore, et cetera. He took care of every emergency and most of the routine chores, all without one word of hesitation or complaint.

I had been proudly showing off my new, very short, natural hair, albeit much grayer than it had been. Now I was going to lose it again. So off I went to the Wig Boutique for a new, grayer wig. This time I wasn't so self-conscious about it. I took my first wig with me and asked for the same style in a lighter shade. I briefly considered going blond but decided that was too great a change, no matter how much fun it might be!

Soon, my hair was so thin that I only went without a hat or wig around the house. When I lost enough hair that I needed to wear the wig all the time, I asked my hairdresser to shave my head again. The first time I had to shave my head, he had stayed after his salon closed to give me privacy from other staff or clients. I was so used to being bald now that this one was only a perfunctory haircut at his regular station. Just think how much money I was saving with only a couple of haircuts a year!

The good news on the family front was that Karen was bringing her boyfriend, Geordie, home for Thanksgiving. We'd met him in May at Stanford and liked him very much. Drew's girlfriend Lynda was coming later in the weekend. Cliff and I were so happy to have all of the kids home at the same time.

For our family pictures at Thanksgiving I wore my gray faux fur hat that Karen gave me for Christmas the year before. It's actually quite attractive — nearly the color of my new wig. But it isn't hair. Here I was, facing Thanksgiving and Christmas again without hair. Two years in a row was almost more than I could bear.

In spite of my physical issues, we all had a wonderful, low-key weekend at home. And Drew made us even happier by proposing to Lynda in December. Their wedding was planned for August 11th, 2001. Hopefully I'd have hair again by then.

KAREN

Thanksgiving was the first time that Drew and Geordie met, and I was relieved that they got along, bonding as they watched football and hockey.

My relief turned to anger when Drew and Lynda got engaged a few weeks later, less than four months after meeting. Geordie and I had been together for a year. I was older than Drew. I knew it was shallow, but I was bitterly resentful of his engagement.

On some level, I knew that my anger wasn't with Drew. I was frustrated that Geordie and I weren't engaged too. When we committed to move to New York together, I was sure that this was our first step toward marriage. I wanted our wedding to come soon to ensure that Mom would be with us. There would be no guarantee now that her cancer was back, but anything we could do to increase the chance of having her at our wedding seemed logical and "right" to me.

I shared my frustration with Geordie — not just once, but frequently throughout that winter and spring. He wasn't ready to make a life commitment and wanted to make sure that when he did so it was because of me and us, not due to external pressures. I appreciated his integrity and understood his feelings. But, the thought of having Mom absent on my wedding day haunted me.

In other ways, Geordie was making incredible concessions in supporting my family situation. He wanted to spend Christmas with me and knew that I wanted to be with my family. So, he came to Virginia that year. It was the first Christmas he celebrated away from his family and I appreciated his parents' generous understanding of his choice.

Lynda came up to Arlington for a few days during our visit and I saw how happy she and Drew were together. It seemed that their heads were always right together, as if they were sharing a secret. If they were apart, then they were looking at each other from across the room, smiling intimately. He had adopted manners that I never knew he had — opening the door for her and helping her down the step of his huge Ford pick-up truck. My parents welcomed both Geordie and Lynda seamlessly into our nuclear family.

Much as this Christmas was magnitudes better than the prior year, cancer still joined us as an unwelcome extra guest. It was Mom's second Christmas without hair. Her chemotherapy treatment seemed to be working — her CA-125 had dropped 30 points to 84, but the side effects were severe and the schedule was grueling. In addition to losing her hair, she had painful rashes on her hands and feet that caused her skin to peel off. The neuropathy in her hands was almost crippling. She couldn't open a bottle of water or even thread a needle to sew.

After its initial drop, her CA-125 had plateaued. The doctor had reduced the dosage to mitigate the side effects, with the reassurance that it would still be an effective dosage.

From what I could tell, she still had most of the side effects, without improvement in her CA-125.

Christmas was my tenth trip home since Thanksgiving the prior year for Mom's surgery. Thank goodness for frequent flyer miles!

I still felt guilty living so far away, but my visits back East helped. So did the multiple times each day that I spoke to and emailed with my parents. I usually called when I first got up in the morning, plus various other times throughout the day.

My other long-distance help strategy was indirect. The prior year when Mom had needed blood transfusions to elevate her platelet levels, I'd tried to see if I could donate them to her directly. The timing never worked, so my second year in business school I decided that I would donate platelets vicariously.

For cancer patients like my mother, transfusion of these donated blood products was critical for surviving chemotherapy. I donated as frequently as I could and hoped that I was helping cancer patients in California as donors in Virginia had helped Mom.

Donating platelets was dramatically different from the typical blood drives I'd participated in. In a two-hour process, the apheresis machines took blood from one of my arms, ran it through a machine that separated out the platelets, and returned the remaining blood to my other arm. Since both of my arms were occupied, I usually watched movies on the personal television attached to my apheresis chair.

My mid-story plea is that if you, the reader, are someone who can bear needles and enjoys a reason to spend a few hours watching a movie in the middle of the day, please consider donating platelets. Donations save lives and the apheresis process helps us understand the countless hours that cancer patients spend with needles in their arms or medi-ports for treatments and transfusions.

My next visit home that winter was for my 28th birthday at the end of January. Actually, the premise of my visit was my birthday, but I had an ulterior motive. I was increasingly worried that Mom's CPA career was too taxing (pun fully intended) combined with her chemo regimen. Since my first priority was for her to survive cancer, I went home with the goal of convincing her to quit her job.

I had my list of reasons as ammunition. She'd already proven that she was capable of re-entering the workforce and succeeding among younger colleagues. She had risen quickly through the ranks of her firm. She had multiple interests outside work — sewing, gardening, and volunteering — which would keep her busy. She needed a break from the rigorous commitments of her office. She'd proven that she could handle work plus cancer, but work wasn't helping her recover.

What I had underestimated was the extent to which Mom's identity as a successful CPA helped her to cope with her new identity as cancer patient — which was clear from the way she spoke about her job that weekend. "I spend so much time relying on the advice of medical experts to deal with my cancer and relying on you and Dad to take care of everything else. When I'm at work, I get to be the expert, and my clients and colleagues rely on me."

I had a new appreciation for why she was unwilling to let go of her career. For all that her job was demanding, stressful and tiring, it was also a welcome distraction from the demands, stresses, and fatigue caused by cancer.

VICKI

Initially, the Topotecan appeared to be successful, dropping the CA-125 slightly. But after the first series, my CA-125 just kept going up. Each month I asked the oncologist to change me to something else, but he kept saying, "Just hang in there. We need to let it run its course."

After six cycles, my CA-125 was all the way up to 154. At that point, he decided to switch to Taxol again, because it had worked so well before. I wasn't so sure it had worked well before, because after all, I still needed chemotherapy! This Taxol treatment would be once a week for three weeks and then one week off — for twelve cycles, or forty-eight weeks. My hair wouldn't come back until I finished.

I planned to attend all four of Lynda's bridal showers, and give her a tea at our house to meet my friends. We were so excited about adding Lynda to our family that the wedding planning provided a much-needed boost to our lives. Cancer seemed to take a back seat, and I was delighted with that. Still, my great regret was that when I was intro- duced to Lynda's extensive family and friends, I was sure I presented the picture of an elderly mother of the groom. No matter how many times I lose my hair, I miss my eyebrows and eyelashes the most. A hat or wig can make up for the head of hair, but nothing can really replace facial hair. I feel so old-looking when my eyes are bald too.

GRADUATION
February – June 2001

Shortly after Christmas, Drew and Lynda began house hunting in earnest. They wanted to buy a house in Mathews, preferably with a few acres of land. They worked with a local realtor and looked at most of the three bedroom houses for sale in the county. They also looked at land that might be suitable for building. Finally, one afternoon Lynda and Drew simultaneously found the same ten acre lot advertised on the Internet and were thrilled when they were able to negotiate a reasonable price for it.

Meanwhile, they also chose a modest house plan that provided for additions later if they wished. By April, the builder broke ground and the great Greve house project had begun. This was quite an ambitious undertaking for two young adults who had known each other for less than a year and had never owned a house.

Cliff and I went down to see Drew and Lynda's property on the day of settlement and continued to visit as often as time and our schedules permitted. We kept taking progress pictures so Drew and Lynda could look back at them years later and enjoy the experience all over again. The project also involved lots of phone calls between us and Drew, and helped to keep my mind off of my chemotherapy and bald head. I am so thankful that they included us in so many phases of their home-building. We both enjoyed watching the house become their home.

KAREN

Much of my family's focus, understandably, was on Drew and Lynda. The house monopolized nearly every conversation I had with Drew or Dad. That spring, I watched my brother grow up. Suddenly, he was making serious financial decisions, negotiating with contractors, and managing work crews — all while working full-time as a high school guidance counselor and planning a wedding. The house took on a life of its own with Drew leading the development.

I struggled to put my happiness for him, and pride in his achievements, ahead of my immature jealousy about his wedding and home plans. It wasn't easy, and I often lost the struggle.

Mom loved her future daughter-in-law and cherished seeing Drew the happiest he'd ever been.

Drew's engagement and house project were also diversions from Mom's cancer. Despite constant chemotherapy, her CA-125 had stagnated in the elevated range of 80-100. She suffered neuropathy in her hands and feet, as well as the indignity of her wig and lack of eyelashes and eyebrows. And then, she suffered the loss of her own mother.

In late February, my grandmother passed away, four days shy of her 80th birthday. Mom joked that Grandma was so stubborn that she would have hung around had she realized that it was almost her birthday. My grandmother had lived a full life, with six children, nine grandchildren and several great-grandchildren, and her body had been failing for decades before it finally succumbed to poor circulation and old age.

A year earlier, I had been with Mom the day she told Grandma that she was sick. She explained to her mother that she had ovarian cancer. Grandma hadn't seemed to understand. Mom slowly lifted her wig from her head, revealing her shaved scalp with patches of quarter-inch hair. Mom and I were both crying, waiting for Grandma's reaction, which never came. I don't think she was capable of understanding that her daughter was fighting a terrible illness. To my knowledge, Mom didn't mention it to her again.

I sat at my grandmother's funeral and prayed for my mother. I prayed that she would live to be the mother of the groom that summer and the mother of the bride at my wedding, whenever that would be. I prayed that she would hold her grandchildren and renew her sewing skills making their little outfits. I prayed that she would see them take their first steps and open presents on Christmas morning. And I prayed that I would be the daughter she needed me to be throughout these experiences.

I tried to time my visits to coordinate with her appointments, but that only covered a few of the monthly doctor's visits she had each year, not to mention the countless blood tests and chemotherapy sessions. She'd been alone for most of her recent doctor's appointments, as she received frustrating CA-125 results while being admonished by the oncologist to "hang in there". It seemed more important than ever that she have support at her appointments. Yet,

I was 2,500 miles away in California. I asked Drew and Dad to make sure she didn't have to go alone, but there was usually a reason why they couldn't go.

The evening before one of her myriad appointments, I asked Mom if Dad were going to see the doctor with her. She said she wanted him to, but he was busy and she wasn't sure if he'd be able to take the time.

"Mom, if you tell him that you need him there, he will make the time. Why don't you just ask him?"

"I hate being the cancer patient who needs to ask for things. I don't want to make him miss work, just to take me to an appointment so that he can hear the doctor share bad news."

"But, don't you want him to be there?"

"Yes, but if it matters to him, he'll go. I don't want to have to ask."

Later, I spoke with Dad. "Dad, are you going to Mom's appointment tomorrow?"

"Oh, probably not. It's downtown and I've got meetings all day in Virginia. Besides, she always goes by herself; she doesn't need me there."

"Dad, I think she does need you there. She doesn't always remember all of the side effects she experiences, and it's got to be hard for her to hear her CA-125 without someone there to support her if it's worse or celebrate with her if it's better. Please promise me that you'll try to go?"

"What time is her appointment … 10:00 A.M.? I can probably fit it in between meetings."

The next morning, I called Dad's cell phone on my way to class to hear about Mom's appointment.

"Hi Dad, how was Mom's appointment?"

"She hasn't called yet — she should be just finishing now. I'm sure she'll call to let me know when she gets to the office."

"Dad, I thought you were going to go with her! I was calling to get the update from you!"

He was immediately put off by my raised voice. His reply was defensive and curt.

"I asked if she wanted me to come, but she said she didn't need me to go with her. I'm not going to skip my meetings if she doesn't want me to be there."

I knew I should back off, but I couldn't. I was furious. "Of course she said she didn't need you. She never asks for help, even when she needs it. That's why I asked you to go. She's had to go to so many of these appointments by herself; I thought you were going this time."

"Well, I didn't and it was because she didn't ask me to. It's over now and what's done is done. We'll just have to wait and get her update later. Now, I have to get on a conference call."

"OK. Dad, I'm sorry I came down on you. I'm just frustrated and I want to be there to go with her, but I'm not, so I can't. I was hoping that you'd go, but I'll just try to get back for the next one." I hung up and stared at the phone. I was shaking with anger and helplessness.

I called Drew, looking for empathy. Wasn't this his responsibility as much as mine?

"Hey Ruf. I'm really frustrated. Do you have a minute?" I downloaded my anger on him and he immediately defended our dad.

"She said she didn't need him to go. So he didn't go. It's that simple."

"But Drew, she did want him to go. She needs one of us to be there with her. I'll be at the next one during my Spring

Break, but can you go to the one in late April? I will have just been there so I know I can't make it back, and I don't trust Dad to go."

"Karen, I can't just take off work to drive up and go with Mom. I went to her early appointments when I was still in Arlington, but now I don't live there anymore. She'll be fine. Really, she's OK."

He was right. He had gone to her early appointments; I hadn't. And she would be fine. But did being there at the beginning absolve him of going to any future appointments? And didn't we want her to be more than fine, but also to feel loved and supported for each step of her treatment?

When I spoke with Mom later, she sounded exhausted. Her CA-125 had almost doubled, from 82 to 154. The oncologist hadn't had much to say besides his typical "Hang in there". I asked her about telling Dad not to go, but she didn't want to talk about it. Either he would choose that it was important to go, or not, but she didn't want to have to beg him. Besides, she'd made it this far going to doctors' visits by herself and she could keep doing it that way.

I felt deflated and distant. Who was I to impose an accompaniment rule on my family if I wasn't available to participate?

VICKI

In April, Karen and I hosted an afternoon tea bridal shower for her high school friend, Anne-Marie, while Karen was home on Spring Break. We asked each of the guests to provide recipes for the book we were giving her and to give a gift of whatever was needed to cook them in. Because of the extensive instructions, and my penchant for doing personal invitations, they took quite a while to write out.

As my May 15th deadline was just around the corner, I wound up writing them in little batches whenever I got a chance. I remember going to a night club to hear Lynda sing during this time. I spent the ride down and the time while we were waiting for her to come on stage busily writing invitations.

This is what my life had become. I could easily have had the invitations printed. I could have had the food catered. But characteristically, and foolishly, I insisted on doing everything myself. Anne-Marie was and is a very special friend of mine as well as Karen, so I was eager to entertain her friends and family. We had a wonderful turnout and enjoyed it enormously.

KAREN

Anne-Marie's mother had abandoned her family when Anne-Marie was just a young girl, and my mother had filled an important maternal role for her since we first became friends. I loved the time Mom and I had that week getting ready for Anne-Marie's tea party. It was the first visit in ages that we'd had fun working on a project that had nothing to do with cancer. Despite interruptions for her weekly blood test — where I saw her nurses for the umpteenth time — and her doctor's appointment — another round of "hang in there"— we had a nearly cancer-free week of activities.

We also discovered that Dad's woodworking skills had prepared him perfectly for the task of cutting paper-thin slices of cucumber for traditional English cucumber sandwiches. The highlight of preparation was making the clotted cream for the scones. Dad couldn't stop saying the words "clotted cream", and with each rendition, "clotted" gained syllables to the point where it became "clah-ah-ah-ah-ahtted cream" in a Dracula-esque voice.

Two months later, Geordie and I went back east for Anne-Marie's wedding. It was a magical, albeit rainy, weekend. That weekend was unmitigated joy for me, watching my best friend marry her love, with the man and parents I love sharing the experience with me.

VICKI

Cliff and I were delighted to attend Anne-Marie's wedding. Throughout her engagement, Anne-Marie had told me about the wonderful wedding coordinator, Amy, who was helping to oversee the whole wedding. I watched the way she so capably kept things moving throughout the wedding and reception, and introduced myself to her during the reception. Karen and Geordie weren't engaged, but I was hoping that would change before long and that we would need a coordinator ourselves.

One of the highlights of the summer was Karen's graduation from Stanford Business School. She seemed to really enjoy and benefit from the experience and could now embark on the next stage of her career. The best part was that she'd be relocating to New York with Geordie. Finally she'd be back on the East Coast — in our time zone and less than three hours away by train!

All of us went to Palo Alto for the event. Cyndi and her husband, Eric, flew out with Cliff and me. Drew and Lynda went a day early to get in some sightseeing around San Francisco. That weekend was our first opportunity to meet Geordie's wonderful parents, Vivian and Jeff, and his brother Andy. Amazingly enough, Andy was engaged to be married in August, one week after Drew. We had dinner with them our first night and it already seemed like we had known them forever. They became good friends in addition to being Geordie's family.

We did very little that weekend, except having dinners together and attending the graduation ceremony. I was relieved to have such an open schedule because rest was crucial for me if I was to enjoy the weekend. The hot sun was unrelenting, and straw hats were a must at the Stanford University graduation ceremony in the stadium. After the main ceremony, the Graduate School of Business graduates convened in an outdoor amphitheater where it was much cooler. Karen and Geordie received their diplomas and a special award for graduating in the top ten percent of their class. We were so proud of both of them.

That evening, Karen and Geordie hosted dinner for all of us. It was very nice — especially for me. After a toast, Karen thanked us for supporting her education and then spoke about an independent study project she'd worked on that year. That truly brought tears to my eyes. She said her research was on the relative awareness and funding for breast and ovarian cancers. She also said she intended to continue doing whatever she could to increase women's awareness of the subtle symptoms of this insidious disease. She presented all of the women with an ovarian cancer teal ribbon pin. The dinner was special to me of course because of her thoughtfulness and devotion to the cause of ovarian cancer. But it was even more special to see our daughter in the role of hostess. She had truly grown up.

We returned home, while Karen and Geordie stayed in California to begin their round of summer weddings and packing for New York. Their jobs wouldn't begin until August.

KAREN

Graduation was a perfect ending to the Stanford chapter of our lives. Best of all, Mom was there. Not only was she there, but her CA-125 had come down steadily since April and was 29 for her last test prior to my graduation. Below the 35 threshold! She was almost done with her Taxol chemotherapy treatment and was in amazing spirits. Just months earlier, we hadn't even known whether she would still be with us for this event. All indications were that the next chapter of our lives would be even better than the last.

WEDDINGS
July – August 2001

VICKI

That summer, Drew spent most of his time in Mathews, staying with Lynda's parents to be closer to the house construction — and of course closer to Lynda. Mathews is located at the lower end of the middle peninsula in Virginia, about a half-hour drive to Irvington on the other side of the Piankatank River. So we decided to spend the last weekend of June at Tides Inn in Irvington, because Lynda's first bridal shower was scheduled for June 30th and Drew's birthday was July 1st.

Karen came with us so it was almost perfect. Geordie was attending a bachelor weekend for his brother, Andy. It seemed that lots of their friends were getting married this year. We thoroughly enjoyed hosting Drew's birthday party and included Lynda's parents. We were beginning the experience of sharing Drew with his other family.

Lynda's shower was so much fun. It was hosted in Mathews by relatives on her dad's side, including two of her bridesmaids. I think most of the attendees were relatives too. They were such welcoming women; we really enjoyed getting to know them. The theme of the shower was rooms of the house, which I thought was a wonderful idea. Because Drew and Lynda were both setting up housekeeping for the first time, every room would start out empty.

KAREN

Lynda's father was the youngest of ten children, and it seemed that nearly everyone we met in Mathews was related to her, in some way. We joked that their new house wouldn't possibly be large enough to contain all her presents — her gifts, like her relatives, seemed endless! The day after her first bridal shower, Drew and Lynda were giddy with excitement as they gave me the grand tour of their house-in-progress. It already had the frame structure in place and we walked around where the rooms would be.

Two days later, I flew up to meet Geordie in Toronto to drive the four hours to Restoule, Ontario, where his parents have their summer cottage. Their cottage is the house where his mom was raised — although it now has full plumbing and electricity, unlike during her rustic childhood. A quick walk down the hill took us to breathtaking waterfalls that connected Restoule and Commanda lakes. Geordie showed me how to swim under the falls to sit on the rock seat inside the thunderous curtain of water. It was spectacular, and I told him so as we sat under the falls together.

He replied with a loving smile, "I know. That's why I've always known that the only woman I would ever bring here would be my wife. You know what that means, don't you?"

I couldn't speak, so I nodded, shivering from joyful relief as much as the chilly water. We might not be officially engaged yet, but now I knew we would be.

Part of cottage life was bathing in the lake using natural soap and shampoo. On the fourth day of our visit, I woke up to much colder weather. I lay in bed wondering how I would wash my hair — I couldn't even imagine going into the lake in the fifty-degree weather, but I was meeting some of Geordie's cousins that evening and wanted to be clean.

His mom, Vivian, must have sensed my hesitation and came to my rescue.

"When it gets cold like this, I often indulge in a shower in the cottage. Don't feel like you need to go in the lake today, just because Geordie does." I gratefully accepted her offer and had a brief, but luxuriously warm shower.

I loved the peace and tranquility of the cottage and could have stayed much longer than our five-day visit. But too soon, Geordie and I flew back to California and the reality of our two major summer themes: moving and weddings.

Anne-Marie's June nuptials had followed the scenic vineyard wedding of my friend and former colleague in May. My Stanford roommate, Katie, and her fiancé John were married in Palo Alto on July 14th, just after our movers took our things. A week later, we attended the Lake Tahoe wedding of other GSB friends. With four weddings over, and four left to go, Geordie and I headed east in my black VW Jetta for my first drive across the country.

Geordie spent most of the next week behind the wheel, with me in the passenger seat wondering if the next stop was the one where he would find a scenic overlook to propose. He'd once mentioned that he didn't want to steal the thunder by proposing before our brothers' August weddings, but I was still hoping that he'd surprise me with a ring on our long drive. Numerous scenic overlooks and special moments later, we arrived at my parents, still not engaged.

VICKI

In mid-July, I hosted a tea to introduce Lynda to our friends. We held it on a Saturday so it wouldn't interfere with church. Quite a few of her family and bridesmaids came up from Mathews and Richmond. I was delighted that so many could be here to meet my friends and the mothers of some of Drew's friends. It was a ladies-only event except for Cliff, Cyndi's husband Eric, and Drew who were the wait-staff for the day.

Although Cliff had helped so much ahead of time and the guys did the work during the party, I was just exhausted. The cancer and the Taxol were really enervating for me. My valiant efforts to continue my activities like a "normal" person always fell short. But I was the mother of the groom and I refused to acknowledge how tired I was during Drew's engagement.

I went to Lynda's two showers in July by myself. For the fourth one, Karen and Geordie had arrived from their cross-country car trip on the way to New York so she was able to go with me. The women of Lynda's church hosted this shower. By now I was beginning to remember some of the names and faces of Lynda's relatives. I was sure I would never learn all of them, but would do my best to try. The ladies were so kind to ask about my health without dwelling on it. It was a hot day so I didn't wear either a wig or hat. But I was beginning to be on the fence about going without a wig at the wedding. My hair seemed to be thinning more each week. Hair loss is one of the guaranteed side effects Taxol has on me.

KAREN

The Monday after Lynda's final bridal shower, Geordie and I took the train to New York and spent the afternoon walking around our new apartment, deciding where everything would go. The next day, the movers arrived with our furniture and boxes. Geordie and I discovered that we are a terrific moving team.

While I arranged the bedrooms and kitchen, he put together the self-assembly pieces of furniture that we'd bought at Cost Plus and IKEA and also set up all of the electronics. Our first night in New York, we'd already unpacked more than I thought we'd accomplish the first week. By the time Geordie left on Friday for Drew's deep sea fishing bachelor party, we were fully unpacked and just a few shopping excursions away from being completely settled.

Enter Mom for the weekend!

VICKI

Karen had told me she wanted me to come up to New York to visit often, and I began those visits much sooner than I had anticipated. The afternoon of the third, I was on the train to New York for what turned out to be my first monthly visit.

We did a few moving-in activities like choosing a new rug for the living room and installing shower curtains. But, Karen also made appointments for us at Elizabeth Arden's Red Door Salon on Fifth Avenue. A cosmetologist named Ernesto applied my make up while coaching Karen on how she should do it for me on the day of the wedding. My greatest vanity was that I looked old with no eyebrows and no eyelashes. I was beginning to develop real sympathy for alopecia patients who go through their whole lives with no body hair. It was still new to me and I was extremely self-conscious.

Ernesto did a wonderful job and I went home armed with a new cosmetic kit full of all of the products he had used. I was sure Karen would remember his techniques and I'd be a very normal looking mother of the groom the next week.

KAREN

A week later, the pressure was on me to create the same effect for Drew and Lynda's wedding activities. On three separate occasions — the bridal brunch, rehearsal, and wedding itself — we laid out her new cosmetics on the dressing table in her room at the bed and breakfast. Mom prepared her face with lotion, foundation and blusher. Then, I meticulously applied three different shades of eye shadow and brushed on eyebrows. I was no Ernesto, but my makeup artistry improved over the weekend and even with my amateur skills, his techniques made a huge difference. The impact of eye-defining shading and liner brought Mom closer to her striking chemo-free appearance.

VICKI

I worked at the office only a couple of days the week before the wedding. We left on Wednesday for Mathews. Our family had booked the entire bed and breakfast called Buckley Hall. Cliff and I had stayed there several times and loved its beautiful antique décor and welcoming proprietor. It was almost a home away from home and served as a great headquarters this week for the groom's side of the family.

Wedding week turned out to be sweltering with the threat of thunderstorms. On Thursday night, Drew joined us for what would be our last dinner as a nuclear family of four. On Friday, we attended Lynda's bridal luncheon hosted by her aunt. Then, Cyndi and Eric arrived in time for the rehearsal and dinner. Suddenly the wedding seemed so real.

As we were hosting the rehearsal dinner at a restaurant, Cyndi agreed to go early to make sure that everything was set up. Our theme was Hawaiian since Drew and Lynda were planning to honeymoon in Maui. I hadn't realized how much I had come to rely on Cyndi for all sorts of moral support and really missed having her at the rehearsal. As Cliff was Drew's best man, and Karen and Geordie were in the wedding party, I sat alone in the first pew. I think my tears began when the pastor gave the initial prayer before even starting the actual rehearsal. They didn't stop until it was over. Fortunately for me, Cyndi would be sitting with me at the wedding.

KAREN

On their wedding day, Lynda was a princess bride complete with glittering tiara, and Drew made a dashing groom. After a tearful rehearsal, Mom was dry-eyed and smiling for the wedding itself. I was a bit tearful at the ceremony and was so grateful that Drew had asked Geordie to be a groomsman and had assigned him as my escort for the recessional.

A furious August thunderstorm provided increased drama for the event, threatening as we were leaving the church. My favorite moment came between the ceremony and reception when Lynda and Mom were walking together toward the car. Drew called out from behind them, "Mrs. Greve!" They turned around together — Mrs. Greve of thirty-four years with Mrs. Greve of thirty minutes. I now had a sister for the first time in my life — and I couldn't have asked for a more vibrant and loving addition to our family.

Geordie flew directly from nearby Richmond to New York for work on Monday, while I planned to spend a couple more days in Virginia. Dad drove home the next day, with Mom beside him in the passenger's seat while I perched in the middle of the back seat, leaning forward to hear each other easily. As we talked about various aspects of Drew and Lynda's wedding — the ceremony, flowers, attendants, reception, and the myriad other details involved, Mom and I started to consider the decisions we might make for my own wedding. As we considered potential venues and types of receptions, I could tell that Dad, and to some extent Mom, were starting to see dollar signs in their minds. Dad started to ask what things would cost — throwing out his estimates. Soon the conversation turned from fun to stressful. And I wasn't even engaged yet! At some point, we all agreed to shelve the topic and return to talking about Drew and Lynda's honeymoon plans, Geordie's job in New York, and other easier topics. But the tension remained.

That night, I lay awake thinking about our conversation in the car. I kept replaying the one aspect of my wedding that no one had mentioned: Mom had been at Drew's wedding.

I had no idea when Geordie would finally propose or when we would be married. None of us had any idea how Mom's health would be. For Drew's wedding, her CA-125 was below 30 and she had a reprieve from Taxol. But we'd seen before how quickly her CA-125 could escalate. I tried to imagine my wedding without her there, and couldn't. My throat constricted and my face felt flushed as I pictured myself selecting stationery, flowers, and my dress with a friend or Aunt Cyndi instead of Mom. I felt nauseous at the thought and tried to push it from my mind so I could sleep. Just as I turned over, I heard soft footsteps walking down the stairs.

I come by my insomnia honestly. As I heard Mom filling the teakettle with water, I put on my robe and slippers and walked downstairs.

Mom turned when she heard me enter the kitchen. "I'm sorry Karen; did I wake you up?"

"No, I couldn't sleep either. I'm just not clever enough to admit it and get out of bed until I hear you. I just keep thinking about our conversation in the car today."

"Me too. And you know, it really upset me. I'm worried that you're only focused on the materialistic aspects of your wedding. What about the people — Geordie most importantly?" She paused as she filled her mug with water, gesturing to another one for me. I nodded and we fixed our tea in silence, my response on hold until we were seated at the table.

As we sat down, I knew what I wanted to say, but had no idea how to say it.

"Mom, that's what I was awake thinking about. I felt trapped in the car talking about the practical aspects of the wedding that aren't the most important part. The most important thing is that I've found the person I want to spend the rest of my life with. Geordie is so much more than my dreams of who my husband would be. But, even though I know we will be engaged one day soon, we aren't yet. And that is driving me crazy. I know I should be patient, but I don't feel like there's enough time."

"Sweetie, you're only twenty-eight. Geordie will propose when he's ready. I'm a little surprised that it didn't happen this summer, but I'm sure you'll have a ring on your finger by Christmas. When you get married doesn't matter as much as knowing that you both want to, and that you've already started planning your life together with your move to New York."

"I know that we will be married one day. But I want it to be soon!" I felt my chest tighten and my face flush as tears filled my eyes, overflowing while I said what had been on my mind for months.

"When I think about Drew's wedding, I get so jealous. Because you were there. You're right that the most special part of our wedding will be having the people we love there. All I care about is that you will be at my wedding. I can't imagine it if you aren't. It's all I think about."

By now, I was blubbering uncontrollably and accepted the Kleenex Mom handed me. She took one herself and mopped her eyes before speaking.

"I know; I think about it too. I'm trying. Being here for your wedding and your children is the reason I endure the chemo, the doctor's visits, the blood tests. Do you think I enjoy all of that? I'm doing my best to be here, but I don't know if I will be. I just can't know."

We reached over the table to hug each other. I felt the tears on Mom's cheek against my own. It was the first moment since her diagnosis when we allowed ourselves to break down together, mutually acknowledging the severity of her illness and our helplessness to control her health.

We slowly separated from our hug when we realized that we were both too congested to breathe. After a cacophony of vigorous nose blowing, we shared our relief at finally talking about the thought that had been foremost on each of our minds. We stayed awake for a few more hours, having the most honest conversation we'd had in a long time — about her health, our frustrations, and finally, doing what we'd started in the car. Now that we'd established that we felt the same about the most important aspect of my wedding, we resumed our conversation about the trivial details that would make it a reality. It was as if we'd made a silent agreement to make sure she would be involved by brainstorming the details prematurely. Ring? Who needs an actual engagement to start thinking about a wedding?

Several cups of decaffeinated tea and half a box of Kleenex later, we ended our conversation with a hug and kiss on the cheek and climbed the stairs to our rooms. Sleep came much easier this time.

VICKI

When we returned to Arlington, I also returned to my Taxol treatments. Probably most doctors would also have prescribed continued Taxol at this point, but I was wondering if I should pursue a second medical opinion. My family heartily agreed and began to exert whatever pressure they could to encourage me to do it.

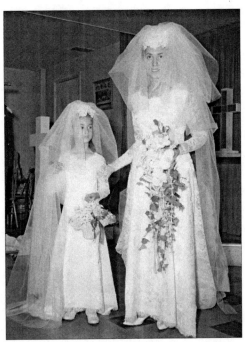

Vicki and Cyndi at Vicki and Cliff's wedding, 1967

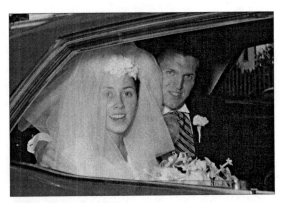

Vicki and Cliff leaving their wedding

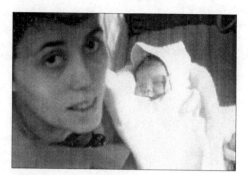

Vicki holding Karen, 1973

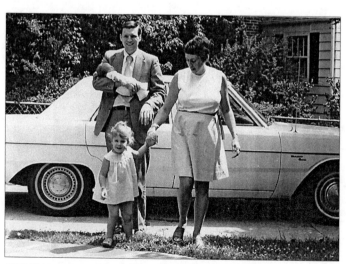

Cliff, Vicki and Karen bringing Drew home from the hospital, 1975

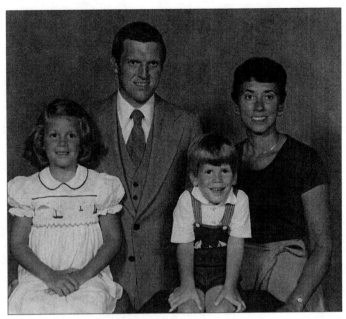

Karen, Cliff, Drew and Vicki, 1978

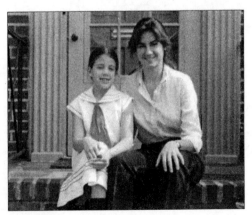

Karen and Cyndi, 1982

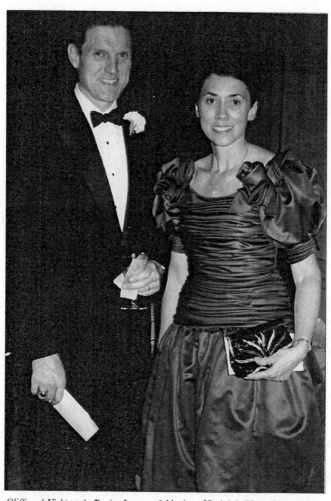

Cliff and Vicki at the Junior League of Northern Virginia's Tiara Ball, 1991

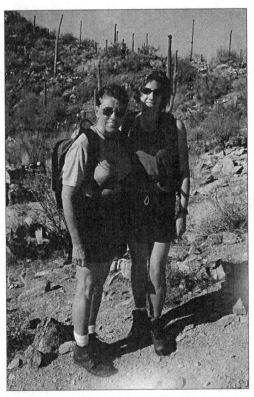

Vicki and Karen hiking at Canyon Ranch, 1999

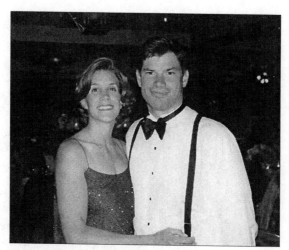

Karen and Geordie at Anne-Marie's wedding, 2001

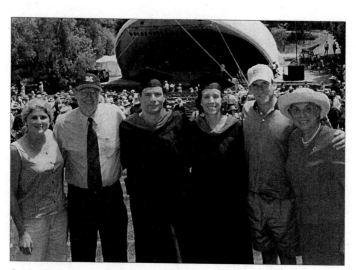

Lynda, Cliff, Geordie, Karen, Drew and Vicki at Stanford graduation, 2001

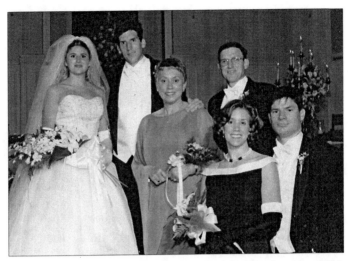

Lynda, Drew, Vicki, Cliff, Karen and Geordie at Lynda and Drew's wedding, 2001

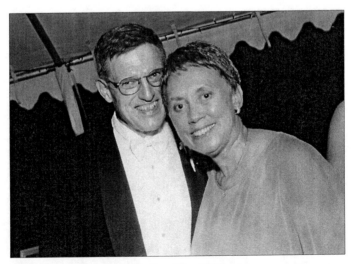

Cliff and Vicki at Lynda and Drew's wedding, 2001

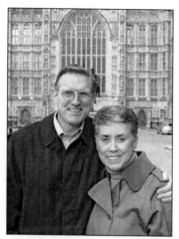

*Cliff and Vicki in front of Westminster,
London, 2002*

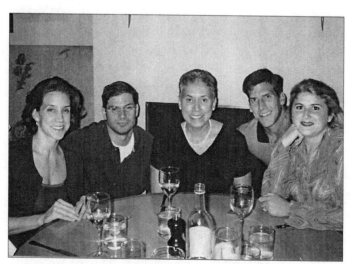

Karen, Geordie, Vicki, Drew and Lynda at a pub in London, 2002

AUTHOR'S NOTE
May 6, 2004

KAREN

Even as Mom and I wrote our story, we couldn't predict its conclusion. As authors, we had no more control over how long our story would be and how it would end than we did as patient and daughter. In that regard, cancer was the main author, its progress hindered by my mother's doctors and treatments, and, of course, her sheer determination to survive.

Tragically, just as cancer gave us the reason to write the book, it subsequently took away the energy, vigor, and finally the life, of my mother and co-author.

It's been seven weeks and two days since my mother passed away. One of my final promises to her was to finish our story and publish our book. To do so, I will have to rely upon her emails and the recollections of friends and family as meager replacements for her voice.

I had imagined that after four and a half years to prepare emotionally and mentally for losing her, Mom's death would be hard but manageable. I was wrong. There is a British expression that perfectly depicts how I feel: "gutted", as if someone has physically ripped out my heart and soul. During my worst moments, I miss talking to her so acutely that I am keening and sobbing and don't know how to stop. This usually happens at night — probably because my subconscious doubts that I could survive these times without Geordie to hold and comfort me. The rest of the time, there's just a dull ache of missing her, even when I'm laughing or happy at the rest of my wonderful life.

Recently, I reviewed what Mom and I had written about the first two years of her cancer journey. I read the sections in Mom's voice and relived talking to her and experiencing those years together. For the zillionth time since I lost her, I wanted to pick up the phone and call her — this time to tell her what a wonderful writer she is and how I admire her bravery in sharing her story. I am acutely aware that, just as my mother's absence has left a gaping hole in my life, the story with her voice limited to emails will have a void as I strive to finish alone what we started together.

TERROR
September 11, 2001

KAREN

Mom sent an upbeat email on September 10:

Subject: Meeeeeeeeeeeeeeeeeeeee!!!!!!!!!

Karen, Cyndi, Lynda (please share with the guys),

Guess my new lucky number is 22!! That is my current CA-125 score — down from 28 which is down from the 3 previous results that were also in the safe range of <35. Now I will truly enjoy our celebration dinner tonight.

I'm not finished with the cancer routine because I need to continue with follow-up tests and visits to ensure the insidious disease doesn't recur. That will be my pleasure. But the weekly treatments are over!

Now the painful part - the DIET (my most dreaded four-letter-word).

Cyndi has agreed to be my daily coach and keep me on track — although all are welcome to assist. I need to lose 30 pounds (yes, it's really 30 pounds) and I know I can't do it overnight. However, I've already started the exercise portion — I've been alternating treadmill with leg lifts for the past 3 weeks. I know that sounds wimpy but it's appropriate while still on chemo. I don't intend to go heavily (pun!) into dieting or weights until at least the end of the week because that is how long it will take my body to recover from this morning's treatment.

... Remember that I frequently find myself on the road at lunchtime and Cliff cooks the dinners — until I can convince him that I'm more than capable again. Also our daily grapefruit for breakfast is now a thing of the past because it disagrees with Cliff's cholesterol medi-cine. (Aren't we a pair!!?)

Your suggestions are much needed and would be very greatly appreciated. If I could look half as good as the three of you, I'd be delirious. Now back to work for me. Thanks for being so supportive of me through all of this.

Much love to all,
Mom/Vicki

As I rounded the 102nd Street crossway in Central Park and ran back toward the 72nd Street exit, I was almost blinded by the early morning light filtering through the leaves. I'd missed deciduous trees during my six years in California: the fresh new leaves of early spring, changing colors in autumn, and lush greenery in between.

It was a spectacular morning. I felt alive and vibrant, overwhelmed by the wonder of life — my life, my love for Geordie, my joy of being back on the East Coast, and my relief that Mom's CA-125 numbers had been below 35 for three months. She might yet be cured! What an extraordinary day to be alive.

It was Tuesday, September 11, 2001.

Two hours later, I was in a morning meeting at my office in Times Square when a manager rushed into the room. "I'm sorry to interrupt, but you all have got to see this," he started, as he walked across the floor toward the windows, "A plane just hit the World Trade Center. You can just see it from the window."

I obediently walked over and my eyes followed his pointed finger downtown. I saw a stream of smoke rising from two-thirds of the way up one of the towers. My colleagues and I murmured our speculation of what might have happened and our hope that no one had been hurt. Our meeting resumed and went for an additional forty-five minutes.

When we were finished, I rushed back through the central corridor of our office to my desk to finish preparing for my 10:00 A.M. meeting. The red light on my phone indicated that I had a message. Actually, as I listened to the automated voice, I had eight. The first one was from Mom.

"Hi Karen, it's me. Please call to let us know you're OK. The news is reporting that terrorists have attacked New York. I'm at the office. Please call me."

I smiled at her melodramatic message. My smile dissipated as I listened to my other messages: from Dad, others from Mom, and one from Geordie. In the month he'd been working at Goldman Sachs, Geordie had never once called in the middle of the trading day. He had called from his cell phone to let me know that he had been evacuated from his offices in the southern tip of Manhattan, but apparently the threat was gone and he was going back to work.

I looked up from my desk to peer around the bay of cubicles and realized that not one of the twenty-four desks near mine was occupied. I heard voices coming from the southeast corner of the floor and hurried over. Our entire staff was there, looking out of the floor-to-ceiling windows at black smoke billowing from both towers of the World Trade Center. A few people were on their cell phones; others were trying unsuccessfully to make calls. Everyone else was silent, listening to the radio news broadcast from the scene.

Moments after I arrived, we watched in horror and disbelief as one of the towers collapsed into itself, releasing a massive cloud of billowing black smoke.

The radio broadcast changed from professional to personal, as the newscasters urged their on-the-scene reporter to leave the site and phone in to the studio. The two male newscasters oscillated between reporting the information they knew of the building collapse, and pleading for their female colleague to call in. She was the first person I realized had died in the World Trade Center tragedy.

I broke from my shocked stupor and rushed back to my desk, frantically dialing numbers into both my work and cell phones — Mom, Dad, Geordie, and Drew — over and over again. I couldn't get an outside line. As I dialed, I read the news on CNN.com. I heard the gasps from my colleagues at the windows and seconds later read that the second tower had also collapsed. A plane had also hit the Pentagon, and online rumors circulated that a bomb had exploded in front of the White House. Dad had frequent meetings at the Pentagon. Mom worked near the White House. How close was Geordie's office to the World Trade Center? I was numb with confusion and concern.

In between my attempts to make calls, my phone rang in my hand.

"Geordie!" I almost shouted into the phone, feeling a wave of relief.

"No, Karen; it's Lynda, honey. Thank goodness you're OK."

Hearing my sister-in-law's familiar, friendly drawl, I felt helpless tears welling in my eyes.

"Oh my God, Lynda. Can you believe what's happening? Have you talked to my parents? Are they safe?"

"They're fine; Drew talked to your mom a couple of minutes ago. Everyone's trying to reach you and they'll be so relieved when I tell them that you're OK." Her tone softened to a question, "Have you heard from Geordie?"

"Not since the towers collapsed, and I should get off the phone so he can get through if he tries to call. Can you tell everyone I'm safe and that I love them?"

"Of course I will. You just take care of yourselves and we'll talk to you real soon. We love you and we're all praying for you."

I pulled out my map of Manhattan to see where Geordie's office at 85 Broad Street was located relative to the

World Trade Center. Six short downtown blocks. I willed my cell phone to ring, while I tried his number from my work phone, again and again.

Finally, I heard Geordie's phone ring. He answered immediately and I felt weak with relief. We hadn't heard from our other New York friends and our focus shifted to them.

I left my office and started walking uptown from Times Square, meeting up with Geordie's Stanford roommate on the walk back to the apartment that Geordie and I shared.

By the time Geordie arrived several hours later, our apartment was full of friends, watching the horror depicted on CNN and sharing our own stories between phone calls and emails to friends and families. We spent the next week home from our respective offices with frequent visits from our friends — comforting each other and watching CNN in increasingly bleak hope that survivors would be found amidst the wreckage.

Incredibly, Geordie and I hadn't lost any of our friends or family members. Thousands of others in New York and around the world were less fortunate. The morning that had begun so spectacularly had turned into the most tragic man-made catastrophe my generation of Americans has known.

The weeks following September 11th were surreal. Almost more so was the gradual return to some sort of normalcy — buying groceries, doing laundry, going to work, and hailing taxis. Any happiness was closely followed by feelings of guilt.

Mom emailed her friends, who had come to be known as the "Second Saturday" ladies, and other friends on September 17th.

Subject: We're all fine

My dear friends,

My apologies to all for being so delinquent in responding …

All in my family and circle of friends are well. Karen's boyfriend was most affected because his office is very near the WTC site. Over the weekend, engineers were in to confirm that the building is structurally sound and the air quality is good enough for the people to return.

We spent the weekend in Mathews with Drew and Lynda. Lynda's brother was the featured star at the family's theatre on Saturday. The show began with a prayer, God Bless America, and the pledge of allegiance to the huge flag that was hung on stage …

Small towns like Mathews, while not directly affected, sometimes react very strongly to national tragedies like the Tuesday attacks. One of the largest industries in Mathews is the D&P Embroidery Company, which makes flags, especially the blue and white star portion of the American Flag. I've never seen so many flags flying as I saw in that little rural area.

Hope you all remain well as we continue to discover how this terrible tragedy will affect us in ways we don't yet anticipate.

Vicki

At a time when people were canceling trips to New York, my parents drove up to visit us. Mom was determined to keep living each day fully and fearlessly. Her perseverance in adverse times was inspiring — and mirrored the overall attitude of courage and oneness that sustained New York City after September 11th.

ROLLERCOASTER
September –November 2001

KAREN

Mom's emails often comprised daily reports of her diet progress:

Subject: Today's number …

… is 164½, which is a cumulative 3 ¾ pound loss so far. I'm thrilled because I am beginning to feel better — largely a result of exercise I think. Kenny the trainer was at the house for the first time this morning. He is WONDERFUL. I hope I still think so after a few sessions although I'm expecting to be a little sore tomorrow. He's about ten feet tall and weighs about fifty pounds. I wish I had a metabolism like his.

If you'll excuse me now, I have to go eat my yogurt and grapes and banana for lunch. Have a great day.

Love you so much,
Mom

_____

Subject: And the winner is ... ME!!!

I've been unbelievably busy for someone who has only about two chargeable hours today. Dad is taking me out for a (diet?) dinner to celebrate my doctor's appointment. So I'm going home in a few minutes and getting on the treadmill. I didn't do my exercises last night because Cyndi was here from six thirty (when I got home from work) until nine thirty when Dad got home. So I hope to do them tonight. Kenny is coming tomorrow morning and then I'm going to the infusion center to have my port flushed on the way to work. Have a client lunch and then nose to the grindstone all afternoon. Hope I can get some free time to talk to you in the meantime.

Have a good evening.

Much love to you both,
Mom

I was so proud of Mom for her exercise and diet — and started to realize that I needed to do the same for myself. I hated getting dressed in the morning and feeling the six pounds I'd gained since business school. Our early October emails focused on our mutual diet goals and frustrations.

Subject: commitment time

Hi!!

I'm really proud of you for your image-consciousness.
But don't overdo it. Remember that you are already
a thin person. Diet if you must, but limit it to favoring
healthful foods over less healthful ones, and portion
control — my worst problem.

I've been a bit of a yo-yo myself re the weight lately.
The only thing that is saving me is the exercise routine.
I gained back more than half of what I lost, between the
weekend (apple crisp, donuts, and wine - not all at the
same time!) and lunch with Cyndi for her birthday on
Monday. As I write this, I'm eating a lunch of banana,
yogurt and fruit cup from the deli downstairs.

… This is an especially difficult week for me …
Tomorrow night we're going out to dinner at the
Cosmos Club with a professional society that Dad
belongs to. Friday night is the Meridian Ball with dinner
first at the Chilean Embassy. Saturday is breakfast with
the girls. All of the events sound wonderful but are
tough on the waistline. At least I still haven't missed any
workouts or treadmill sessions.

… Remember the words of my daughter — don't beat
yourself up about splurges, just concentrate on better
habits going forward. Remember too that there's always
tomorrow (Scarlett O'Hara) to improve.

Have a great day and be kind to yourself.

Love you both,
Mom

On Monday evening, October 15th, I started to open the door to our apartment, but it was locked with the dead bolt. After Geordie opened the door for me, I walked inside to see brown twine crisscrossing our entire apartment. It was wrapped around furniture in the dining area, kitchen and bathroom, and wound downstairs to the living room and upstairs to our bedroom.

Geordie asked me if I wanted to play a game. I dutifully and giddily started following the string. It went everywhere. Within two minutes, I'd kicked off my heels to avoid tripping. Then I reached a piece of paper with a question.

Question 1: What was Geordie's number in junior hockey?

The paper had two holes punched in it with strings leading in different directions depending on the answer I chose: 12 or 18.

This was easy, because it was the number he used on his Yahoo email: 12. I followed the string, to a dead end tied around a table leg! What? He shook his head with a smile — twelve had been his number in midget hockey, but it was eighteen in juniors. I sheepishly went to the eighteen and continued to follow the string around the apartment, answering questions along the way.

Question 2: What is the mass of an electron? $6.26 * 10^{-26}$ kg … 9.11×10^{-31} kg.

I remembered 6.26 * something from chemistry, so I

followed that string. Wrong — I was 0 for two! I was also realizing that I was in love with a geek, but I guess I already knew that.

Question 3: How many players are on the field for one team at one time in Rugby? 15 … 11.

Finally, an easy question. Rugby has 15 players; football has 11. I was one for three.

The questions continued with an assorted mix of Geordie's favorite topics. After nine questions, I'd only answered four correctly. I followed the string to the bookshelf in the corner of our living room for question ten, with Geordie standing next to me. I didn't see string leaving the bookshelf, so I knew it was the last question. I was a little anxious, partly because I didn't want the game to end; I was having so much fun. I also hoped I knew what the last question would be.

Question 10: Will you marry me? Yes … No.

My heart jumped into my throat. I looked at him and I think I said, "Really?" He later claimed that I said, "Are you kidding?" I felt like I was in the best dream of my life.

He'd done it. He'd really surprised me.

I kept hugging and kissing him until he asked if I wanted to follow the string. THE RING! I'd forgotten that there would be a ring attached. Now that I knew I would spend the rest of my life with him, the ring didn't seem to matter.

I started following the string, which led to a copy of Dante's *Inferno* on our bookshelf. Geordie confirmed that I'd said "Yes," right? In my nervousness, I was following the wrong string! At the end of the Yes string was a beautiful diamond ring set in platinum, its brilliant-cut center stone flanked by a smaller diamond on either side.

We called my parents, who were both surprised. Geordie had called my father that day to ask for his approval, but told him that it would be a while before he proposed. Of course, Dad had already told Mom. Keeping secrets were never Dad's strong suit, hence Geordie's quick proposal.

We called Vivian and Jeff next and they welcomed me to the family.

The following morning, I left two messages for Mom during the ten-minute walk between my gym and my office — just letting her know how happy I was and asking when we could talk about wedding planning, now that it was legitimate.

Email banter between Mom and me changed focus from diet to wedding planning, as she wrote:

> ... I have a sneaking suspicion that there are more aspects of wedding planning than either of us realize. For myself, I just plan to have fun.
>
> :) :) :)

Even though Mom and Dad had just visited at the end of September, they came up again two weeks after our engagement. I was embarrassed to admit how much I wanted to show my engagement ring to Mom, and she seemed equally embarrassed to admit how much she wanted to see it.

> Dear Karen,
>
> ... If I could just convince myself that we don't need so much money, I'd scale down my work and leave early enough to actually catch the sunset on my way

home. Sun up and sun down are my favorite times of day! And we spent so much time on our honeymoon watching the sunrise and sunset that I'm reminded of that special time with every sunrise and sunset I see. I don't always want you and Drew to know just how busy I am and how I have to rearrange things to be with you, but it was well worth the hassle and overtime in order to see you and Geordie on the weekend and Drew and Lynda on Tuesday. Spending time with family is and has always been my priority. I hope you'll have the luxury of as much family time as I've enjoyed.

Have a great day.

Love,
M.O.B.

Later that week, I emailed Mom about creating a wedding website for our guests. Her response, signed M.O.B. for Mother of the Bride, showed both her enthusiasm, and the limited time in her jam-packed life.

Subject: website

You are a very clever, innovative, and creative person. Let me know what you decide to do. My only suggestion about your web address is to keep it as short and as simple and easy-to-remember as possible. Have a great day!!

Much love,
Your 20th century mother (aka M.O.B.)

Even Mom's emails that weren't about the wedding had some wedding element. For instance, F.A.B. was her email nickname for Cyndi: Favorite Aunt of the Bride; B was my nickname as Bride.

Subject: New low !!!!

Dear Coaches (B and F.A.B.),

This morning my weight was a new post-cancer low of 162 ¾. Although it's a long way from my ultimate goal, each day's goal is just to be lower than the previous day. So, I've met yesterday's goal and it's only Tuesday. I generally improve as the week goes on so hopefully this week will be no different. More later. Must earn my keep.

Much love to you both,
M.O.B.

Geordie's mom was scheduled to visit us the first weekend in November, coinciding perfectly with our trip to look at reception sites in Washington, DC. I was excited because I wanted her to feel like part of the wedding planning process and I knew from Mom's experience that the mother of the groom misses out on much of the wedding planning, no matter how hard the bride tries to keep her involved.

We drove down Saturday morning and spent the weekend at my parents' home. It was a whirlwind of showing Vivian a bit of Washington, while visiting three potential reception sites, meeting with the pastor, and connecting with Amy, Anne-Marie's wedding planner.

By the end of the weekend, we were all exhausted, but we'd decided on a date — October 12th, 2002, hired Amy, and selected the reception venue that was everyone's favorite — the Washington Monarch Hotel. It was lovely, with an open courtyard and airy-feeling atrium for pre-reception cocktails and a clover leaf-shaped room with a raised dance floor in the center for dinner and dancing. It also happened to be just six blocks from our church.

Mom was in high gear working out various details and in the two days after our trip to DC, sent me a series of eight emails with various rehearsal dinner suggestions and details. Her ninth email was back to our least favorite topic.

Subject: CA-125

Cliff, Karen, and Cyndi,

I'm truly sorry to send you such a dismal message. Six weeks ago, the CA-125 was 20. The test from Friday spiked to 108. The doctor was so surprised that it was repeated today to ensure it was done correctly. No matter what the new result, I'll be having the test done every two weeks for the next few months. He is inclined to wait to resume Taxol until after the holidays - January. I told him how important it is to me to have hair for Karen's wedding, second only to the importance of actually being at the wedding. He was surprised that I feel so well. His comment was that he is treating the patient, not the test number. If I really feel this well, he thinks it is appropriate to wait until after the holidays to resume treatment.

Given my penchant to look on the positive side, if you would have been inclined to toast my good result today — had I had one — I encourage you to instead toast the fact that I am still beating my one in three odds and will continue to do so until this wretched disease is gone for good.

I'll keep everyone posted with the new test result, etc, but please don't call to talk about it today. I'm pretty upset and have quite a lot of work to do before I leave at my REGULAR time. Cyndi, I'm more resolved than ever to take off the weekend for the quilt retreat. I'll be ready to leave whenever you are on Thursday. Please keep this undercover at the retreat. There's no point in distressing lots of folks when I don't know how bad this is yet.

Have a great day all.

Love you so much!!
Vicki (aka M.O.B.)

After she sent the update on her appointment, she shared her email back and forth with Dad, starting with his reply to her CA-125 email.

I won't call, but I want to say that I love you. I'll get stuff for dinner on the way home and pick up your prescription, and try to be there when you get home. See you tonight.

Love, me

I'd like to work out before dinner and will try to get home early enough to do that. This time I'd like to begin chemo thinner and more svelte!! People will be so bedazzled by my figure and size that they won't notice that I don't have eyelashes.

:) Keep smiling.

I love you

Aren't those the nicest emails from your dad?! I'm much better this afternoon. I'm going to be in the office until around five thirty when I'll be heading for home. Call any time but I won't be able to talk for long because I have so much to do — here and at home.

Love,
M.O.B.

I was stunned when I got Mom's emails. We'd thought she was in remission; could this be a mistake? I felt the familiar nauseous feeling of hearing a bad test result, compounded by the fact that, once again, Mom had been alone when she'd received bad medical news. The only silver lining was the dialog between my parents. Dad's thoughtful emails brought out Mom's positive attitude — she was telling him to keep smiling by the end of their banter! Her optimism was incredible, which was lucky since the test wasn't a mistake.

Subject: CA-125

The test done yesterday scored 132, up from 108 last Friday. A message has been left for the oncology nurse to call me. Hopefully she'll let me know if the oncologist wants to see me sooner rather than later and if I should start the chemo sooner than January — I'm recommending next week.

How did that song go — "all I want for Christmas is my eyelashes?" Karen, you and I are gonna hafta learn to do the fake ones on me!!

After the second test, the oncologist reacted immediately and decided to put Mom back on Taxol with the now familiar rationale that "it had worked before". But had it worked, when her cancer came back again so quickly? Mom wasn't sure, but definitely didn't want to wait.

Subject: Chemo …

… begins on Monday. Because of the upward trend of my CA-125, I insisted on not waiting until January. The doctor may do an MRI in the next few weeks in hopes something shows up. I've never thought of myself as a model, but the radiology department at the hospital certainly does have lots of pictures of me!! Have a great evening. :)

I talked to Mom several times after her two bad tests, but she seemed to want to focus on other things, especially my wedding. So, I sent her a preliminary wedding budget which received immediate feedback regarding my estimate for her Mother of the Bride dress based on a link I sent her.

Subject: RE: first cut at a budget

… I loved the designer. I loved the dress. I experienced a wave of nausea at the fee — and it didn't include materials …

I'd rather get a less expensive one so we can spend the balance on something else — like transportation back and forth from NYC. I noticed it was missing from the budget but I think it should stay that way. If we added absolutely everything that was even remotely wedding related, your dad would have apoplexy.

Have a great evening. Let's discuss when we have time.

Love, M.O.B.

I laughed at Mom's email about the wedding budget, but couldn't stop thinking about her CA-125. More than anything else, I wanted to be sure she would be at my wedding — whatever dress she decided to wear.

I assumed that her doctor was an accomplished gynecologic oncologist, and that he served most of his patients very well. But, I no longer believed that he was the best oncologist for my mother, and she was the only patient I really cared about. Over the past two years, Mom had frequently expressed her frustration with the oncologist, particularly how she found him to be patronizing and hated his "hang in there" mantra. But whenever I mentioned the possibility of her seeking a second opinion, she countered that she felt loyal to him and believed that he was giving her the best possible care.

When he suggested that Mom start Taxol for the third time, she also became a non-believer. The next day on the phone, she mentioned to me that she was thinking of getting a second opinion. She said that she'd ask her current oncologist if he had a respected colleague with whom he collaborated on patients. I told her that I thought that was a good idea, and tried not to be overly enthusiastic or pushy.

What I really wanted was to get an impartial treatment assessment from a gynecologic oncologist who was not associated with her current doctor or the hospital. As so often happens with Mom and me, she came to the same decision independently, after seeing her therapist that morning.

Subject: Me

Dear Karen,

Carter suggested today that I investigate a second opinion at one of the top U.S. cancer hospitals, and I agreed.

... If you could visit a few websites to get any kind of lead for me I'd really appreciate it.

Love you so much.
Mom (M.O.B.)

Mom finally wanted to pursue a second opinion! Needless to say, Bain lost a lot of productivity from me over the next few days as I got online and researched ovarian cancer resources. This research evolved into a four page letter to my parents. I didn't want to overwhelm them, but if we were finally going to get a second opinion, I wanted to be aggressive and thorough as we thought about our approach.

Several of the world's preeminent cancer centers are based in the United States. Everything I read led me to select one whose extensive medical center and world-class clinical research included a dedicated ovarian cancer research program. So many of the websites lauded their work on women's cancers, and then proceeded to give brilliant examples of their work with breast cancer. I wanted Mom to be at a place where ovarian cancer was an independent focus, not a poor cousin in the women's cancers department. This cancer center wasn't near my parents' home, but I hoped the caliber of the doctors would be well worth the hassle involved with traveling to see them.

I re-read what I'd written, made a few changes, and sent off my email. Mom's reply was almost immediate.

Subject: RE: Second Opinion Research

Dear Karen,

Thank you so much for doing the research for me. Aunt Cyndi is apparently going to do a little research as well. I had an extremely tearful conversation with her last night — she was the only person I could reach — after I spoke with the nurse about just what kind of cancer I have.

... According to the nurse, my diagnosis is "poorly differentiated papillary serous adenocarcinoma." Serous refers to being in the blood system. Poorly differentiated means that it is harder to tackle and more aggressive. I asked her to confirm that I am really only (as if "only" were a good term here!) a stage 3C. She said that yes, I am.

... She has ordered an MRI to include lungs as well as abdomen and pelvis. Although it hasn't yet spread into the lung cavity, her concern and mine too is that the lungs may be where it is headed. The news really hit me badly and I'm not coping with it very well. I'm sorry to be sending this to you in an email but I don't know any other way without losing control at the office — and I surely will lose control if I try to talk about it. I'll try to call you tonight, but may not be able to.

... All of the above notwithstanding, I hope you and Geordie have a wonderful weekend. We will be fine this weekend — in Mathews with Drew and Lynda. The fact that I now know more about my physical situation doesn't change the situation or anything; I'm just more informed. I plan to do some curtain fabric shopping with Lynda and just generally help out where possible at the house.

Much love to you both.
Mom (M.O.B.)

Mom's email about her conversation with her nurse struck a familiar note. I was pretty sure that she'd heard about her cancer's staging before — in fact, I remembered a similar reaction previously. Her email reaffirmed my impression that sometimes she received bad news, became shocked and upset, then forced the negative information to the back recesses of her mind so that it wouldn't impact her daily life and outlook. I think her resistance to focusing on the dismal medical prognosis of her cancer probably helped to sustain her positive attitude, but it was frustrating to hear her get upset again at "new" information about the disease, its staging, or the survival statistics. I fully anticipated getting a similar email in the future after she'd re-forgotten and then re-learned her dire prognosis.

RESOLUTIONS
November 2001 – January 2002

KAREN

When Geordie came home from work the following Friday, I was in our kitchen making dinner. I'd just gotten home from work myself, so I was rushing around making a quick and easy stir fry. Our kitchen was so tiny that I could do everything from one spot — pivoting to the right for the stove and to the left for the refrigerator. I did a full 180-degree pivot to the left to give him a welcome home kiss. He kissed me back quickly, as if he were distracted.

"Hi sweetie. How was your day? Is something wrong?"

"I don't know; you may have to tell me." He inhaled deeply, then turned to get a chair from the breakfast nook and sat in the kitchen doorway. "The head of my desk approached me today about transferring to London, England. It sounds like it could be a great opportunity for me. He actually wanted me to fly out this weekend to meet the guys in London next week. I told him that I couldn't miss Thanksgiving with your family, but could fly there from DC for the following week."

With that deluge of information, Geordie stopped and looked at me. I realized that the chicken pieces I was stir-frying were sticking to the skillet and pivoted back to deal with them. I needed to think a bit before replying.

I loved visiting London and it would be exciting to live abroad for a few years, but would I be able to work there — either by transferring with Bain or taking a new job? How would we plan our wedding from across the ocean? How much better was the London desk than the one in New York where Geordie was working now?

Amid these other thoughts and questions was one that drowned out the others. I'd seen Mom at least once each month since moving to New York, and with much greater ease than our nearly monthly visits when I was in California. I wasn't ready to move even further away in the other direction. Mom's cancer had taught me how precious time with her was; September 11th had expanded this lesson to include my entire family and closest friends.

I took a deep breath and turned back around to share my thoughts and concerns. He said he wanted it to be our joint decision, and was unwilling to even consider it if I said I didn't want to go. But the more we talked, the more clearly I saw the life reality that it would never be a "good" time to uproot ourselves — and in future years, our family — and move across the ocean. Plus, he'd gotten clear signals that this opportunity could accelerate his career. Likewise, refusing it could backlash against him.

We spent hours over the next few days discussing "the London thing" and weighing its pros and cons until we'd thought through a full list of questions for him to take with him on his trip.

I was petrified to tell Mom about our potential transfer, and certainly didn't want to share the news on the phone. My instinct was to tell her in person when we were back for Thanksgiving that weekend, but I didn't know how. I decided to share it with Drew and Aunt Cyndi, so they could help me think through the best way to approach Mom. We decided to wait until after Thanksgiving Dinner, so as not to spend the entire meal talking about it.

I was nervous throughout dinner, and felt deceitful talking about our jobs and wedding plans without mentioning London. I was also horrified to realize that everyone around the table — Geordie and me, Drew and Lynda and Aunt Cyndi and Eric — knew about London, with the glaring exception of my parents.

I served everyone their choice of apple, pumpkin or pecan pie, and then shared our big opportunity. My parents were stunned to hear that we might be moving to London, but this paled in comparison to Mom's reaction to being the last to know. She felt hurt and betrayed that I'd shared such potentially life-changing news with everyone else before sharing it with her, exacerbated by the realization that she'd had us all around her Thanksgiving table for hours with everyone else knowing as she sat oblivious to the tidal wave about to break.

To her enormous credit, Mom was able to distinguish between her personal hurt feelings and the decision at hand. She was unilaterally supportive of our opportunity. She had been to London twice and had thoroughly enjoyed both visits. Between her passion for gardening and love of formal afternoon tea service, she was a true Anglophile. In contrast, with his love of the great outdoors and hunting — not the

British sport of going after foxes with horses and hounds, but the American version of man with rifle following deer and turkey — Dad was a bit mystified why anyone would move to London. Of course, Dad never would have chosen New York City either.

On Sunday, Geordie left for London and I returned to New York. On Monday, Mom returned to scheduling medical appointments. Aunt Cyndi shared one of Mom's emails with me, her response to my aunt's offer to go to her next MRI appointment with her in an email signed "Your pushy little sister".

Subject: Today

Dear pushy little sister,

This has been the most marvelous day — following two days so dismal that I left early and took a nap before dinner both days ...

I'd be honored and touched to go to my MRI with you. It's scheduled for Wednesday, December 5th at noon ... I'll be spending the morning at a client's and will hotfoot it home to meet you. Unless you'd rather meet me at the hospital — your choice.

Your grateful seasoned sister,
Vicki aka M.O.B.

Geordie's visit to London exceeded his wildest expectations. He marveled at London's open space relative to New York's claustrophobic skyline and was impressed by the traders he met on Goldman's London desk. The only negative was that he'd been misled about the financial package associated with the transfer. Often, transfers from US investment banks enjoy luxurious "expat" packages. Not so for a junior trader in the fall of 2001. My intention had always been to try to transfer my Bain position, but now I had to for financial reasons.

I kept Mom up to date on all of the details as we got them.

Subject: RE: good morning

Your life is almost too exciting for my weak heart.
Thanks for sharing the info with me. Please send me
Vivian's email — unless you have already. I'd have a
better shot at communicating with her via email than by
snail mail. Have a great day.

Much love to both of you.
Mom (M.O.B.)

Amid London and medical second opinion planning, the wedding provided a stress diversion. Mom and Aunt Cyndi came the first weekend in December to see a couple of Broadway shows and shop for wedding gowns. Our trip to a cavernous wedding dress destination in Brooklyn confirmed the dress selection that we'd made over Thanksgiving weekend in DC. Our wedding was starting to feel real, as was the staggering cost that it would entail for my parents. For the next few weeks, Mom and I talked at least once every day — usually more like three to four times — and emailed several times daily during the week. Our emails were almost completely focused on London logistics and the wedding — budgets, photographers, dresses, and musicians.

At some point in our back and forth in the second week of December, we also set our medical plan of action. The referral nurse at the cancer center outlined the two different options for pursuing second opinions and offered us four different appointment times between December 31st and January 7th. I shared these with Mom and she replied almost immediately.

Subject: RE: second opinion trip

My preference is Monday, January 7th, because the week before will be a short week anyway and we can fly down on Sunday ... also, it should be my week off chemo. Thanks for taking care of this!!

Love you,
M.O.B. :)

Dad emailed me separately.

Subject: RE: second opinion trip

Thank you so much for doing this for Mom. Even if the cancer center agrees that what the oncologist in DC is doing is optimum, it will give Mom confidence that she is getting the proper care. If it turns out that there are other courses of action, it might really change the course of events.

Love you, Dad

It was a huge relief to have the appointment scheduled, and to have Dad's support for what I was doing. I was as hopeful as he was about having her seen at a world renowned cancer center and the opportunity to make informed opinions about her doctor's approach. In my heart of hearts, I secretly hoped that the cancer center would recommend a miracle treatment option — a different chemo, radiation, or clinical trial — that would put an end to Mom's miserable cancer roller coaster.

The last I'd heard was that my Bain transfer looked "more likely than not", but I wouldn't know for sure until January 7th — the day of Mom's appointment. Geordie needed to tell Goldman whether he could start in London on January 21st. We decided to take the plunge; if my transfer didn't come through, I'd job hunt in London and cross my fingers.

As January approached, my desire to go to the cancer center with Mom started to be overwhelmed by my stress about our impending move to London. Mom was understanding when I said that I just didn't think I could get away to go with her. Both Dad and Aunt Cyndi would go with her, and, in her words, there was no need for a huge entourage! She solicited our input before they left.

Subject: cancer center

Karen and Cyndi,

As you both know, we leave on Sunday for my appointment at the cancer center. I'd appreciate your developing a list of questions you think we should be prepared to ask. Be as creative and thorough as your time permits. Hopefully, we will remember to ask about all the relevant issues, but I'd rather have the crutch of your suggestions. Thanks in advance.

:) Me

I was amazed at how Mom was engaging in her medical care and I shot back a list of various topics to ask about with questions outlined for each: medical treatment options and side effects, diet and exercise, diagnostics for tracking results, the continued role of the cancer center in her care, and the possibility of participating in BRCA1 or BRCA2 genetic testing.

Subject: RE: cancer center

Thanks! You are a wonder! After this is all over, you and I are going someplace nice to celebrate — and I don't mean just dinner.

Love you so much,
Mom (M.O.B.)

When I suggested that we throw ourselves a party on October 12th, 2002, and even knew a great venue and band, she countered.

Subject: cancer center

October 12th definitely belongs to you and Geordie!! You and I will do something totally separate and prob-ably later when we are sure I'm out of the woods —

which I am determined to be eventually!! Hold that
thought. Thanks for all of your help.

Love you,
Mom

The world renowned cancer center lived up to its repu-
tation — if anything Mom's experience vastly exceeded our
hopeful expectations. Mom underwent another CA-125
test, MRI, and pelvic exam. Then they met with one of the
cancer center's gynecologic oncologists, a young doctor with
excellent credentials. Mom had worried that the appointment would be difficult with so many voices in the room,
but apparently everyone was sensitive to making it work,
so it did. Mom asked the primary questions, with Dad
augmenting. Aunt Cyndi held back from participating —
except to take copious notes — until they seemed finished,
then added her own insightful and helpful questions.

The process after my family returned to Virginia was
almost as impressive as the visit itself. Once the MRI and
CA-125 results were available, the cancer center oncologist they'd seen met with others in his department to discuss
the best treatment options for Mom. The review committee
included clinical oncologists, radiologists, and surgeons, so
that the approach would reflect options in all disciplines. We
nervously anticipated our Friday conference call in which he
would summarize their recommendations.

He and his colleagues recommended that Mom start
on Doxil, a second line chemotherapy which had shown
positive results with other ovarian cancer patients. They
thought it best to cease Taxol for the time being and gave a
rationale that made sense to all of us. Apparently, when a

chemotherapy works once, it may also work in subsequent treatments. However, it is most effective to leave significant time between treatments of the same therapy, so the cancer doesn't build up resistance to the therapy.

The cancer center oncologist was happy to have Mom's primary care remain in DC and to consult with her local oncologist and review Mom's progress regularly. This was a huge relief to my mother, and to all of us. We'd finally taken the necessary step of confirming Mom's care approach and had high hopes that her health would improve with the benefit of the cancer center's expertise.

TRANSITIONS
January – March 2002

KAREN

Our relief at having forged a new, multi-expert approach to Mom's care was short-lived. As willing as the cancer center's oncologist was to collaborate, the local oncologist was equally resistant to coordinating with "a young, inexperienced oncologist". He suggested that if she wanted to pursue a second opinion, he'd arrange a meeting with one of his local colleagues. He never blatantly refused to change the treatment protocol to Doxil, as the cancer center had recommended, but he was nasty in his dealings with Mom.

After hearing about her first appointment back with the local oncologist, we made sure that Dad, Aunt Cyndi or I accompanied her each time she saw him. I think we all hoped that she'd exaggerated his bullying — and were shocked to find that the opposite was true.

In the meantime, Bain approved my transfer and the timing worked perfectly — I finished my case in New York in January, but the London office wasn't prepared for me to start until March. I emailed my schedule to Mom, to see when we might schedule wedding-related appointments during my transition period.

Subject: RE: the latest and greatest

What an exciting and upbeat message!! At the moment my calendar is completely open. Given that I have Carter on Tuesdays at noon and Kenny on Thursdays, either Monday or Wednesday would be best for me. The only other complication for me would be chemo, which is generally Monday, but I have no idea now what the schedule will be by then. Actually, Wednesday is also a quilting meeting and you are welcome to go with Cyndi and me if you like.

Have a great day!!

Love you,
M.O.B.

This email from Mom in which she expressed her enthusiasm at being completely available, and then mentioned that she had other commitments four of the five days, plus her full-time career, was a perfect reflection of how she lived. She was frenetically busy, but determined to fit in the activities that were most important to her, which usually meant all of them.

In mid-January, Geordie flew to London and I went to my parents'. At my first visit with the oncologist, I was much less reserved than Mom. When he made his first backhanded comment about the cancer center oncologist, I quickly responded that we'd been overwhelmingly impressed with the interdisciplinary approach at the cancer center and felt it imperative to work with a doctor who was willing to collaborate to seek the best treatment alternative. He replied that he would recommend a local second opinion if that was so important to us, implying that we'd hear the same things he told us. I quickly countered that our goal was to find a separate and independent opinion — to which his reaction was sullen.

On the way home from that appointment, I asked Mom if she'd mind if I spoke with the cancer center oncologist about recommending another local doctor. I just hated for her to have to deal with her first oncologist's attitude, and was fearful that the benefits of having an extra perspective would be wasted if we continued with him.

At first, she didn't want me to. The local hospital was really convenient for her office and she felt loyal to the medical team she'd started with.

Her loyalty waned when her CA-125 nearly tripled from 122 in early January to 345 on February 1st. I urgently emailed the cancer center oncologist to ask how soon we should see improvement from Doxil and whether he could refer a local doctor who would be more receptive to collaborating with the cancer center team. He recommended that Mom do three courses of Doxil before expecting to see a significant decrease and reconsidering the treatment. He referred us to a gynecologic oncologist who had done her fellowship at the cancer center and whose office was near my parent's home.

A few weeks later, Dad would accompany Mom to her first appointment with the oncologist recommended by the cancer center. For all of Mom's loyalty to her former oncologist and his team of nurses, the new oncologist and her team's professional approach confirmed the decision to change. She actively collaborated with the consulting oncologist from the cancer center, so we felt that we had a world-class support network deciding Mom's care. Even if Mom hadn't been convinced of the need to change before she made the switch, her decision was soon validated. A few months after she left his practice, Mom's original oncologist left the local hospital for a private practice that was not at all convenient for her.

In the meantime, during my extended winter visit, Mom and I had several wedding-related appointments each week — for the invitations, bridesmaid dresses, florist, photographer, and other details. She raced from chemo appointment to office to meeting to wedding appointment. She invariably brought work home at the end of the day, but seldom had the necessary energy to work in the evening. Her fatigue had become progressively worse with each chemo regimen, and now was really debilitating.

Beyond fatigue and hair loss, each chemotherapy had its own unique set of debilitating side effects that challenged Mom's ability to function. For Taxol and Topotecan, the greatest problems were her skin rashes and neuropathy, but she managed to cope and work around them. Doxil's side effects were proving to be more of a challenge. In February, she'd had flu-like symptoms that led to rapid weight loss and a struggle for energy. Worse, her feet and hands swelled and became chafed soon after she started the treatment. She began to get terrible blisters that made it difficult for her to even put on shoes, much less wear them for more than a few steps at a time.

This was an added insult to my mother as shoes had always been a weakness of hers, which she attributed to her difficulty in finding a comfortable fit for her size 10AAA feet. When she first discovered Salvatore Ferragamo, she had found a friend for life. Even back when she and Dad were starting out — in the days when going to McDonald's for dinner was a treat — she would scour the sales rack at Neiman Marcus and buy herself a pair each year. She now owned a collection of over thirty pairs of Ferragamo's, all carefully maintained in their original boxes.

By early Spring, she was reduced to wearing slippers everywhere, including the office. She kept her most comfortable pair of Ferragamo's under her desk for client meetings, but otherwise exchanged calf leather for fleece. Even so, her feet developed terrible blisters, as did her hands from writing and typing.

Something had to give, and she finally decided that it was her career. She was clearly torn about leaving KPMG and I tried to be as supportive as I could. I reminded her that, after a 20-year "maternity leave", she had returned as a second year tax specialist and flown through promotions to the highest non-partner position in the firm. Her clients adored her and her colleagues depended on her. She had maintained her professional standards while undergoing chemotherapy for two years. My stance was that she had nothing left to prove.

Then, we discovered that she would actually make more money on her disability than on her salary, since disability is two-thirds pay, untaxed, and her tax rate was greater than thirty-three percent. It eased her stress about leaving work when she realized that it wouldn't have a financial impact.

Mom officially gave notice on February 18th after she got an even worse CA-125 test than the one two weeks earlier. Her email to Dad, Aunt Cyndi, and me indicated her resolve.

Subject: Me

We made a good decision over the weekend — it's definitely time to move on. My CA-125 was 379 this time. Also, my kidney function was borderline dangerous. The good news is that the red cells and white cells are good enough to have chemo tomorrow. Meanwhile, I'm spending my time catching up and cleaning out at the office.

... Have a great afternoon and thanks for always being there.

At the end of February, I left DC to join Geordie in London. I spent my first days walking around the city and trying to acclimate myself to my new home. I had flown over for a few days in January to find a flat for us to rent, but otherwise, I had only been to London twice. The architecture was as beautiful as I'd remembered. The weather was worse than on my previous visits. It rained constantly — not a cleansing, refreshing downpour, but an incessant, frigid drizzle. My umbrella and I became close friends as I learned to navigate between other pedestrians on the sidewalks by tipping it one direction or the other between competing black shields.

Since I had a few days before work and we didn't move into our new flat until the 20th of March, I went to visit my Harvard roommate Victoria in Leiden, Netherlands, for a few days. She took a break from researching her Ph.D.

dissertation to show me around the town and take a daytrip to Amsterdam. I don't think we stopped talking — sharing stories, thoughts, and feelings — for three days, except for brief breaks for food, wine, and sleep.

When I returned to London, I appreciated another aspect of Victoria's close proximity. She was my only friend whom I could call before midday. The earliest I could call Mom was noon my time; which was seven o'clock in the morning her time. Likewise, she couldn't call me after five in the evening, as I usually went to bed by ten. As the spring progressed, this made me selfishly grateful that she was leaving KPMG. I was looking forward to talking to her during the day without worrying about making her job even harder by taking time away from her clients.

Subject: Flowers

… I received flowers yesterday at the office from the Controller's office at one of my clients. People are so amazing. So many folks have wished me well that I can't change my mind now and stay on …

Have a great day!!

I think the hardest part of leaving KPMG for Mom was leaving her colleagues and clients. I was impressed at how supportive most of them were — sharing words of encouragement and sending flowers. Of course, not all were so gracious and a few colleagues grumbled that "they'd like to take time off work." I'd like to think (but doubt) that she responded in kind by suggesting that maybe they'd like to use that time for chemotherapy treatments!

Her team at KPMG shocked her by hosting a going away tea party at the office one afternoon. She was still excited and a bit tearful that evening when she called to tell me about it.

"I was already having a hard enough time holding myself together, when Randy blew me away by giving me a gift on behalf of the team. They never give going away gifts to anyone but Partners! It's a Baccarat crystal star paperweight engraved with KPMG's logo and then my name and years at the firm. I can't wait to show it to you; it's so special and my description can't do it justice. I already have it on my desk at home."

It was bittersweet for Mom to leave the career chapter of her life, and we were all concerned about helping her transition. With our dad out of town for her final day, Drew made a huge effort of driving three hours to take her to dinner, and then driving back three hours to work again the next day. His email confirmed my concerns.

Subject: Greetings from Mathews

Hey Karen,
I haven't talked to you in forever! I'm glad to hear through email that it seems like you are really enjoying London. I'm really glad to hear that. Any big change like that is usually tough to adjust to, and you've done it quickly. (Do you realize that you have now lived in four of the world's major cities?)

Anyway, I don't want to write another Mom email, but I always want to stay updated and I know you do too. Because Friday was her last day of work, and Dad was in St. Louis, I went home Thursday to have dinner with her. I don't want to say she was different, but in a way, she kind of was. Everyone at work was treating the party like a "going away party", but not going away from work, but going away from life. Apparently, Mom feels like she's being treated like she's going off to die. When I responded to her (to try to make her feel better) that it wasn't like she was going to die in a week, that she was just going on disability so she could enjoy the finer things in life for a while, like orchids and quilting, and that she was at an appropriate retirement age, she replied that no, she was terminally ill, and just couldn't work anymore.

When we got to the restaurant, I offered to let her out at the door on a night with perfect weather, thinking she would say, "No, I'd love to take a walk with my son," but she said, "Yeah, I'm really tired these days and my feet hurt, I think I'm going to take you up on that." I didn't want to write this to depress you in any way, but I've kind of had a rough time since I saw her and my mind is constantly preoccupied (not that you need this distraction in a new job in a new country). I just want to keep the communication open and give you as many updates as possible since you've been so great at updating me.

I guess what I'm trying to say is that I was hoping that going out on disability would help her a lot, and in the long run it probably will, but for right now, it seems like her spirits are kind of down.

… I asked my boss if, from time to time, I could go up to see Mom when Dad was away on business and she replied that it would be fine if I counted that as sick leave. So I'm going to have to budget my visits carefully since I've only got a very limited number of sick leave days, but I'm going to try to visit more.

Anyway, sorry to ramble on and on so much, but I did want to talk again and this seems like the easiest way. Hope you and Geordie are both doing well. I can't wait to see you all again. I hope you're having a great day.

Love you,
Ruf

MOTHER OF THE BRIDE
April – October 2002

KAREN

Mom never experienced the void she'd feared when she left work. Her days remained busy with doctor's appointments and treatments, and now she was able to spend the rest of her time with friends and family at an easier pace. In her own words, her decision to go out on disability was "long overdue". She had too much going on with planning a wedding and fighting cancer to spend her days at the office.

Part of Mom's adjustment was to do her living at a slower pace than before. Because of her fatigue and blistered feet, this was less a choice than a necessity. At least her CA-125 was responding, plummeting from 345 in February to 116 in April.

She and Dad came to see us in London for Easter, eight days after Geordie and I settled into our new flat. The family joked that she'd fallen off pace. In New York, she came to visit me within two days of our moving in. Soon after they arrived on Thursday, Mom and I went out for a bit of shopping around our neighborhood. Dad had warned me in no uncertain terms to minimize the walking, but I had no idea how serious her blistering had become. After walking for less than five minutes, she confessed that she really needed to go home and take her shoes off. When she did, blisters covered the backs of both of her feet — about the size of a quarter on one heel and twice that on the other. The bottoms of her feet were bright red and puffy.

At least, for once, I felt equipped to help her. After rowing crew for eight years in high school and college and then running marathons in my twenties, I was a veritable blister expert. She looked away as I used a sterilized needle to drain the fluid from each blister to help them heal and be sure they wouldn't rupture.

Mom took a nap after our medical adventure, while Dad and I went for a walk/run to Hyde Park. He was annoyed with me about Mom's feet, but conceded that it was almost impossible to do anything meaningful without injuring her delicate skin.

We discussed our increasing concern about Mom's doctor's appointments. She tried so hard to maintain her positive attitude, that she would forget or downplay her symptoms during appointments. I'd seen it during various visits to her former oncologist and it was happening enough with the new oncologist referred by the cancer center that she had become reluctant to sign Mom's medical disability forms for work. When the doctors would ask Mom how she was feeling, she would reply that she was a little tired, but OK. She would mention specific symptoms — neuropathy, blistering, and rashes — but downplay the impact they had on her daily life. She'd completely forget to mention other aches and pains unless they were happening on the day of the appointment.

Both Aunt Cyndi and I had repeatedly encouraged her to start keeping a journal of her symptoms and feelings. She even had at least eight or ten lovely journals at this point, from us or various friends and well-wishers who wanted her to be able to write about her experience and feelings. But she didn't use them, and really, I couldn't blame her. She was so busy trying to cope with her symptoms that she didn't want to spend her time writing about them too.

So, Aunt Cyndi and I had started sharing her symptoms with each other. I felt more than a little guilty at first about having these side conversations about mom without telling her, but the purpose was to help her get the best possible care — not to exclude her or scheme behind her back. During our outing, I asked Dad to do the same, and to tell me honestly how things were so we could work together to advocate for Mom's health.

The next day, Mom and I started a tradition. I bandaged her blisters and called a taxi to take us to Claridge's Hotel for tea. She wore her most comfortable "real" shoes and then discretely took them off under the table while we indulged in a proper English Afternoon Tea. We sat in the luxurious foyer for over two hours, starting with a champagne toast to her newly "retired" status and my new home. Mom always toasted something at restaurants, even toasting her CA-125 when it got worse — that it wasn't even higher. The afternoon flew by as we sipped tea and champagne and talked about my wedding, London, and her retirement.

When I was fourteen, Mom had taken me to my first

ever Afternoon Tea during our family vacation in London. She showed me how to split the scones and then to enhance them with clotted cream and jam. It was one of her first times at tea as well, and even as she taught me, she subtly peered at adjacent tables to be sure she was doing it "right". In retrospect, knowing how many ladies at fine London Afternoon Teas are tourists just like we were then, I suspect that others may have been checking out her technique at the same time.

Fifteen years later, our second Afternoon Tea at Claridge's Hotel marked a different first. It was the first time ever that she let me pay the check. I'd been thinking for days of a persuasive rationale for paying. When the check arrived, I quickly grabbed it and reached for my credit card. The expression on Mom's face was a funny combination of annoyance and indulgence.

"What, exactly, do you think you're doing?"

"Well, you've treated me to numerous wonderful afternoon teas over the years. Now that I live in London, the home of Afternoon Tea, I've decided to start a tradition of taking each of my lady guests to fine tea during her visit. You're my first guest, so we're starting the tradition." I hoped I sounded more confident than I felt. I had tried to pay for numerous things and meals over time and had never won this game.

She wasn't giving up easily this time either. "I think that's a wonderful idea and I hope your other female guests enjoy it. I know that I'll especially enjoy this Afternoon Tea after you give me the check so I can pay."

So, I decided to try the pleading tactic.

"Please, Mom. I'm nearly thirty years old, with a good career and stable income. I really, really want to treat you for once. You've always taught me to be generous with my friends and family, but you never let me be generous with you. I promise that when we go out to other meals, and even tea in the States, I won't argue about the check. But I want to establish a precedent for paying for tea when we're in London."

To my happy surprise, she acquiesced — eyes brimming with tears. "I'm so proud of you and the woman you've become. I graciously accept — but only in London."

She and Dad left on Monday morning. After my parents returned home, Mom and I continued to talk at least twice daily, mixing phone calls with emails about wedding details. By now, we'd made most of the big decisions: date, venue, band, flowers. I don't think either of us had fully appreciated how many details went into creating the wedding we'd both dreamed of having.

We were also surprised by another aspect of planning. We discovered with relief that we had similar visions for the day, from the aesthetics to the scope and quality of everything we did. We had minor differences, but they were insignificant compared to the stressful wedding tensions my friends described with their parents.

In May, Mom came back to London for her second visit in two months, this time with my Aunt Cyndi. Swimming upstream amid the crowds of British and international garden enthusiasts at the Chelsea Flower Show, Aunt Cyndi and I were relieved that Mom was able to walk along with us, albeit slowly. We lamented at the vendor tents that the only one of us who lived locally was also the only one of us without a garden, or even a window box, in which to use the various planters, tools or horticultural specimens.

Later that visit, Aunt Cyndi's jaw dropped when Mom acquiesced to let me treat both of them to tea. She applauded me when she heard the "rules" I'd successfully imposed, to which Mom quickly responded, "Don't get any ideas!" When it came to financial matters, she had a tendency to treat her kid sister much as she did her kids — "treat" being the operative word.

Just four days after Mom and Aunt Cyndi flew home, I was on my way to Virginia myself for my bridal shower hosted by Mom's friend Nancy. We had a four-day holiday weekend for the Queen's Golden Jubilee, celebrating her fifty years on the throne.

On Tuesday after my shower, I went to Mom's oncologist appointment with her. The doctor made it clear that more information is better than less, especially when it comes to Mom's side effects. She wanted to know about everything, even if we thought it may not be chemo or cancer related, so that she could judge.

Based on Mom's skin reactions, she decided to reduce the Doxil dosage in the hope of mitigating the side effects without losing the therapeutic impact. She wanted to stay with Doxil for at least two more cycles. Mom's CA-125 and other tests were steady, so she thought that the Doxil was keeping the tumors at bay for now.

Dad went to Mom's next doctor's appointment with her and reported by email that her CA-125 had inched a bit lower yet, to 116! That was a good thing, because Mom was much too busy wedding planning to cope with bad cancer news. Each time she emailed me with details, like this email about my bridesmaid dresses, I felt lucky to have her in charge of the wedding logistics.

Subject: Budget and dresses

Dear Bride,

Thanks for the budget. I'll update it manually and give you the changes — I'm too cyber-challenged to try to update it on the computer by myself!!

I picked up your shoes at the bridal shop today ... I didn't pick up the bridesmaids dresses or pay the balance while I was there. The dresses are really pretty. The stoles weren't with the dresses and I assumed they would be shipped to the girls. When I asked about them, the staff person found them in a separate place. Each was wrapped separately in cellophane and the first one I looked at had poorly done corners ... They agreed to fix them but if they still don't look good enough, I'll fix them myself. Thankfully we have enough time ...

I also booked my ticket to London for the July trip this morning. I'm so excited about coming. Hope it really won't be too much company for you. Dad insists he will be so busy with work there is no way he can come any time this summer. I'll probably be glad to be out of his way and won't be that much missed. Good thing this message is to you and not Cyndi — my syntax is terrible.

Have a great day!!

Love you so much.
M.O.B.

In July, Drew and Lynda came to London to visit for a week. I had to laugh at Drew when they arrived to see me at Bain their first day, after walking over from our flat.

"Everyone's so nice. A couple of people asked if we were Americans and offered to give us directions if we needed them. How do you think they could tell we were tourists?"

I looked at my brother in his John Deere tractor cap, shorts and rowing t-shirt, backpack and running shoes. He was so endearingly rural American. My friends, parents, and even Drew and I, always marveled that we'd grown up together in the relatively cosmopolitan suburb of Arlington, Virginia, and then gone in completely different directions. I jumped from major city to major city whereas he had moved permanently to a small town. He had even completely adopted a rural Virginia drawl, whereas I was starting to add British intonation and vocabulary to my neutral accent.

Drew and Lynda practically walked through the soles of their shoes as they explored London, also taking in a side trip to Dublin. I think the highlight of their visit was going to see *My Fair Lady*. Lynda had recently starred in their local performance of the musical and she loved seeing the professional version in the actual Covent Garden setting of the play.

The highlight for me was when Mom joined us for the end of their visit. It was so hard to get all six of us together. This time, Dad was the one missing, but usually it was Geordie. Again, I got to treat my family ladies to tea, although Mom hesitated a bit before letting me pay this time given the recent frequency of our tea splurges.

Dear B,

I had a fabulous time. Given how much time I slept, it's amazing that I also did so much while I was in London. You are a wonderful hostess and the best daughter a mother could ever dream for ...

Have a great day!!

Much love,
M.O.B. (and so happy about it!!)

A week later, Mom got her new CA-125 result. Even though it was stable at 129, she was really demoralized that it hadn't gone down.

Subject: My appointment

This week's health news could have been a lot better all the way around!!

As you know, my CA-125 was 129, up from 116 last time, which was down from 129 the time before. My oncologist referred to it as "stable."

Cliff wasn't able to go with me to the doctor because of his proposal. However he was able to work efficiently enough to come home two and a half hours earlier than he has been. At least he got some down time finally. So, here are my best recollections from the visit.

Although I didn't realize it before (it wasn't ever mentioned on the MRI reports) my oncologist said I actually have three tumors: the left groin tumor is slightly larger than before, the right groin tumor is slightly smaller than before, and the vaginal tumor that I was unaware of is unchanged or slightly larger.

She is recommending that I have round eight of chemo tomorrow. Then, depending on the results of the next MRI, she may either resume Doxil for two more rounds or wait until October to change to something else. Either way, it is a decision point. I reminded her that we agreed with the cancer center oncologist to contact him at the next decision point and she was supportive of that …

I told her I didn't want to change to anything else until after October 12th and she agreed after I explained (wedding hairdo and eyelashes).

That's all for now on the medical front. Thanks for your interest and continuing support. This certainly does seem like a long ordeal to me.

I knew from talking to Dad that he had made a huge effort to get home early to be with her after her awful appointment; meanwhile, Mom was clearly frustrated that he was able to get home early, but hadn't taken the time to accompany her to the appointment itself. Fortunately, her disappointment didn't keep her from fondly remembering their wedding on their anniversary the next day.

Karen,

... I talked to the calligrapher this morning. I'm picking up the envelopes on Monday. I think it's entirely appropriate that I work on mailing your invitations on our 35th anniversary. I can't think of a better way to spend the day. I promise not to let my reminiscing get in the way of quality control!!

Have a great evening.

Love you so much.
Mom and M.O.B.

Geordie and I went back to see my parents in August for our final pre-wedding visit. Mom and I had all of the usual meetings that characterized my recent visits home, plus others that Geordie needed to attend as well. Our wedding was starting to feel close and real.

Our appointment at the bridal boutique was my first dress fitting. I couldn't believe how beautiful it was — the full length sheer veil was edged with the same delicate lace that adorned the bodice and hem of the porcelain silk gown. Mom's eyes filled with tears when I put on the gown and veil together for the first time and turned to show her.

On Sunday, Geordie's parents joined us for a dessert engagement party that my parents hosted to introduce Geordie to about thirty of their friends. Drew and Lynda came up from Mathews too, so we had both sides of our new family all together except for Andy and Blanca.

Geordie's parents, Jeff and Vivian, stayed after for a few days to visit with my parents. It was Jeff's first time to the area. As a retired high school principal, he likes to know his surroundings, and preferably to be in complete control. Within a few days, he was proudly navigating the streets like a local.

Meanwhile, Geordie and I had to get back to work and took the red eye flight back to be in our offices bright and early Tuesday morning. I stared jealously at him on the flight home. He always managed to sleep six of the seven hours of a night flight, versus the two to four that I slept under the best circumstances. This time I was particularly keyed up after all of the excitement of the visit and the realization that it was our last trip back before our wedding in October.

I was also worried about Mom. She'd underplayed her recent doctor's appointments, but I kept thinking about her three tumors. When I was home this time, Mom showed me the two on either side of her groin area. I could actually feel the hard, matchbook-sized masses under her skin, as she could every day when she dressed or undressed — or just felt for them under her clothes.

The next week her CA-125 went up to 200, indicating further growth of the cancer. Mom tried to downplay her concern, but she was clearly worried, as was I. Together, her local oncologist and the cancer center oncologist decided to continue her Doxil treatment through October, partly because of Mom's desire not to lose her hair before my wedding. It seemed certain that she'd meet her primary goal of being at my wedding, and I couldn't blame her for wanting to look her natural-haired best on a day that she'd spent months planning for and years dreaming about. I hoped that the positive energy she was spending on the wedding would help both her spirits and her health, and not exhaust her to the point of making both worse.

Over the next five weeks, Mom and I talked on the phone even more than usual and emailed back and forth multiple times each day about the myriad details. As RSVPs started to arrive, she also sent me daily updates of who would be joining us for our wedding, and who was unable to attend. Just a few of Mom's emails give a taste of what our month was like…details and excitement galore!

Good afternoon Bride,

I'm sitting on the edge of my chair waiting for additional guests to respond via mail. So far we have cards for 21 with no real surprises. 197 RSVP's to go.

Have a great day, and thanks for letting me have such an active role in your wedding. I told you we would have fun doing this!!

Love you so much,
Mom (aka M.O.B.)

———————————

Subject: More acceptances 8/31

Dear Bride,

… We are now at 58 attending, 8 regretting. My little box of cards is getting full.

Thank you so much for the nice note you sent about the party, et cetera. I think Dad and I enjoyed it as much as everyone else did. Except that I am so exhausted that I have slept-in most days since.

Hope you had a wonderful weekend full of celebrating. Have a great day!

Love you so much,
M.O.B. (and social secretary for the future Mrs. Young)

_____

Subject: Today's snail mail

Dear Bride,

We got only two cards today - both "Yes" with nice messages: "and can't wait!" and "Thank you for this kind invitation. We can't wait to join you in celebrating Karen & Geordie's wedding."

Truth to tell, I can hardly wait myself. We are now at 96 "Yes" and 22 "No" - about 81%. You and Geordie are much loved by so many people.

I just don't understand why people wait so long to respond. Don't they know I'm sitting on the edge of my chair watching for the mailman each day?!

… Have a great day. This is really fun!

Love to you both,
M.O.B.

Subject: Bridal Brunch addresses

Dear F.A.B.,

It is my understanding that the bridesmaids, mothers, aunts and, of course, bride, get invited to the bridal brunch. I'll provide their addresses and Karen can confirm — given that she has time — I realize she just whiles away most days staring at her lonely engagement ring, longing for the day when it gets company. Isn't that what this is all about? ...

Thanks so much again for doing the brunch. It is a huge amount of work on your part, but will be greatly appreciated by all attendees, especially Bride and me.

M.O.B.

Subject: Fwd: wedding stuff — what else?!?!?!?

Dear Bride,

I just got your lovely voicemail message that REALLY, REALLY, REALLY made me cry! I have an idea I'll be doing a lot of that in the next few weeks — yes, extending beyond the wedding. The other day, when Dad was teasing me about having his lines memorized (when the pastor asks, "Who gives this woman?" Dad replies, "Her mother and I"). I told him he may need to learn to say instead, "I do," because I'm not sure about giving you away. I prefer to think of it as just gaining Geordie and his family instead of losing you.

Don't know what brought all this on this afternoon because I've been so steady and calm and full-speed-ahead about everything until now. I remember that when Aunt Carolyn got married, I spent the week before the wedding at the Greve's (then unrelated to me). I was fine until Friday night. Right after the wedding I started to cry and I didn't stop until after I went home at the end of the weekend. Hopefully my emotions for your wedding will mirror my emotions at Drew's and not Carolyn's wedding. Can you see the headlines? "Happy couple leaves for honeymoon in Mauritius right after Bride's mother is checked into hospital for traumatic response to nuptials."

Have a great day! I'm available to talk and sew except between three and four this afternoon when I get my manicure and haircut. More later.

Love you,
Mom

_____

Subject: Re: Insomnia

Dear Bride,

I'm sorry you couldn't sleep last night and I wasn't available at midnight my time to talk to you. I'm off to Carter now, and will give you a call when I get home. If I lose track of time, call me before you go to bed.

Love you two so much. More later.

Very happy and excited mother of the bride

BRIDE
October 2002

KAREN

I was giddy and excited as I cleared U.S. customs on the Sunday before our wedding. I walked through the electronic doors and scanned for my parents among the cluster of family, friends, and car service drivers waiting for passengers. There they were, smiling mischievously as Dad held aloft a large white sign, with "BRIDE" printed in crimson letters. Wow, it was really happening!

Something else was happening that week in DC — something terrifying. In the car, my parents shared the latest details about a horrific local crisis that had begun just four days before. Six people had been shot and killed in two days by someone now known as "the Washington Sniper". So far, all of the attacks had been either further out in Virginia than my parents' home, or on the Maryland side of DC, but I was more than a bit concerned about having all of my closest friends and family come together in DC amidst such a crisis. My parents showed the same pragmatism and resolve they had after September 11ᵗʰ. We certainly couldn't stop living our normal lives just because of a madman over whom we had no control. The best way to "win" was to proceed as normal, in this case with my wedding.

The next morning, Mom and I set boxes of goodies along the dining room table and worked our way down the assembly line to make hotel welcome bags for our out of town guests. Mom had amassed quite an assortment of food and gifts: bottled water, maple leaf cookies (to honor the Canadian contingent), Virginia peanuts (for the Virginia counterparts), Ghirardelli chocolates (for California, where we'd met), DC maps with a list I'd compiled of worthy sights and activities, a schedule of the weekend's events, and finally playing cards imprinted with our double dogwood wedding logo. Aunt Cyndi had designed the logo when she learned that the dogwood was both the state flower of Virginia and the provincial flower of Geordie's native British Columbia.

Geordie arrived Wednesday evening. I was relieved to have him there for the last few days before the wedding. I'm not sure he felt the same way, given the mad final preparations underway, but he had plenty of his own errands to do in preparing for the Friday men's golf outing. The balmy, relaxing golf day he'd envisioned was proving elusive. Weather reports predicted heavy rains on Friday morning. More threatening than rainclouds, there was another sniper murder on Wednesday at a gas station en route to the golf course.

We all strove to focus on the wedding and ignore the sniper crisis, but it wasn't easy. The day before our wedding, I had planned to go to the gym before the bridal brunch at Aunt Cyndi's. I was about to head out the door when I hesitated and changed my mind. The only common threads to most of the sniper attacks were that they were at or near gas stations, and were close to freeway entrances. The Gold's Gym I went to in Arlington was next to a gas station about two blocks from the nearest entrance to I-66. I imagined the headline, "Arlington woman shot one day before her wedding" and abandoned my workout in favor of a quick run on my parents' treadmill. There was another attack that day, but it was at a gas station an hour away.

A frigid torrent of rain came down throughout the morning. To their credit, Geordie's friends and family — including Dad and Drew — stuck it out through nine holes in the torrential downpour. I assume they had plenty of beer to keep them warm. Meanwhile my bridesmaids, Aunt Cyndi, Aunt Carolyn, Vivian, Mom, and I were cozy in Aunt Cyndi's living room sipping mimosas and eating quiche, dutifully served by Eric. I think the rain eased his disappointment of being stuck helping with the ladies' bridal brunch instead of playing golf with the guys.

We returned home to hear Drew and Dad describe their golf morning. It sounded even soggier and colder than I'd envisioned. The sloppy conditions probably contributed to the 5-way tie for first place, out of five foursomes. Drew and Dad played with Clint, Geordie's best man and a single digit handicap golfer, and came out winning the tie breaker.

As our wedding approached, I tried to stay relaxed, but my calm façade was starting to crack. Mom sat with me while I finished getting dressed for the rehearsal dinner. Just having her there calmed my tensions. She looked radiant. She was wearing a dark grey silk dress with hand painted tree branches and birds, with a matching scarf around her long neck. Mom zipped me into my rehearsal dress, a pale yellow silk slip dress adorned with a cascading watercolor floral bouquet.

"You know, I didn't like that dress when you first bought it, but now I think it's perfect. You look lovely."

"You're so funny! I knew from the first time I showed it to you that you didn't like this dress, but you insisted on pretending you did. I don't know whether you really like it now or not, but you just made me feel much better." I paused. "You're sure it's OK?"

"It's perfect, like I said. Let's go rehearse."

We met Geordie and the rest of the bridal party at the church. He looked dashing in a new blue shirt and yellow tie I'd bought him in London. I stole him away from the group for a little kiss.

"I missed you today. I love you so much. Can you believe this is really happening?"

"Yes, I can. Are you ready?"

I was ready, although I knew my nerves were still right on the surface. Dad practiced walking me down the aisle and lifting my veil at the end, before I grabbed Geordie's hand and stood with our wedding party at the front. I was starting to grasp the approaching reality of our wedding and I didn't want any of it to end.

Before we left for the rehearsal dinner, Reverend Wimberley called all of us together for a few brief words.

"I hope everyone feels comfortable with what'll be happening tomorrow. You all did great tonight and it's going to be a wonderful ceremony. Now, I want everyone to try to remember something. This is a wedding. It's a stressful event and things may go wrong with some of the logistics — it is part of the experience. But over the next twenty-four hours I hope you'll remember the most important aspect of the day.

Each of you is here because Karen and Geordie love each other, and they love you, and you love them. I hope you'll be able to think about that as stresses arise and remember the reason you're all here celebrating."

His speech was exactly what I needed to hear. That was the point of everything, wasn't it?

The tables at the rehearsal dinner were adorned with American and Canadian flags, set amid paper maple leaves in fall colors. Geordie's dad welcomed everyone to dinner — handing out tiny Canadian flag pins so we could all be honorary Canadian citizens for the evening. Our meal flew by, with toasts and roasts from our friends and lively conversation at every table. The best story came from Victoria. As a Fulbright scholar now studying in Belgium, she'd been invited to a dinner at the King's residence. As it happened, the dinner was scheduled for the evening of our wedding. So, she wrote him, "Dear King, Although I am honored to have been invited … I must decline, as I have a prior engagement for the wedding of one of my closest friends . . ." Victoria is originally from near Liverpool, England, and told the story in her Americanized Scouse accent to peals of laughter from all of the guests.

By the time our toasting, roasting, and gifts were done, I realized that it was just after nine thirty, the time for which we'd invited the rest of the guests for cocktails in the bar area! Sure enough, I rushed over to find a group of Mom's friends already there. Within an hour, the bar was humming with an eclectic assortment of our friends. It was a good preview for us of how overwhelming the next day would be as all of our worlds converged in one wonderful party.

As much as I wasn't ready to end the evening, by eleven thirty, I was completely exhausted. I also finally noticed that

Mom looked about twice as tired as I felt, despite her cheerfully strained smile. Geordie stayed to keep the party going
as I left with my family for home. The next time I'd see him
would be at the end of the aisle at our wedding ceremony.

Exhaustion overcame excitement and I slept most of
the night after our rehearsal dinner and party. Dad and I
met downstairs Saturday morning for our ritual commentated run up Mount Post Office. Whenever we did this
three-mile route, we exchanged running commentary as we
approached and passed the "summit".

"The elder Greve is nipping to the inside of the turn as
they approach the peak. He's holding strong, but now the
junior Greve is coming up on his left after darting around a
parked car. It's nip and tuck as they approach … and, again,
the result appears to be a tie." This was the last time we
commentated our race as Greve-Greve, and it was a fittingly
momentous start to the day.

Later that morning, our house was transformed into a
makeshift beauty parlor for several hours, as my bridesmaids,
Mom, and I walked around at various stages of preparation — some bridesmaids with full makeup and natural hair,
some with hair in an elaborate up do and undone morning
faces. By mid-afternoon, we were all ready and left for the
church, taking our wedding clothes to change in one of the
church classrooms.

I paced nervously while everyone started to get dressed.
Soon, all of my bridesmaids were dressed and looking
gorgeous, as was Mom. We'd found her dress months before
and she'd really resisted buying it, since it was much more
expensive than most of her evening dresses. It was a heavy
silk dress in a luxurious dark silver color, with a matching
jacket that closed with a crystal Pavé-style clasp. It looked

so stunning on her that I'd practically begged her to buy it and she'd reluctantly agreed. It was so typical of her to be willing to spend a fortune on my gown, but then be budget-conscious for her own.

Finally, it was time for me to get dressed. I felt like Scarlett O'Hara before the ball as Mom helped me with the clasps to my corset and Blanca attached my stockings to the garter belt hooks. After I slipped on my garter (with a blue ribbon), another bridesmaid tied my crinoline around my waist. Finally, about six sets of arms helped to lift my wedding gown over my head without messing either the dress or my hair and makeup. Mom and Aunt Cyndi carefully lifted my full-length lace veil and securely anchored the comb under my headband. The hairdresser had especially adorned the white fabric headband for me using lace and pearls left over from Mom's wedding gown, which she'd made herself thirty-five years earlier.

Just after I was dressed, Reverend Wimberley came in to review the vows with me. Wow, this was real! At a quarter to five, we all left the room. Dad and I waited in the hallway during the processional music for Mom and then the bridesmaids. Then, suddenly, I heard the wedding march and we started down the aisle. My heart pumped with happy nervousness as I saw row upon row of our friends and family and looked ahead to our wedding party and Geordie. Geordie looked absolutely overcome with emotion. His chin quivered as he struggled to maintain his composure amidst the magnitude of the moment. As soon as Dad lifted my veil over my head and kissed my cheek, I stepped forward and grasped Geordie's hand. We looked at each other and felt an electric calm pass through our firmly clasped hands. This was so exactly right.

Throughout the ceremony — the readings, Reverend Wimberley's lesson, and Lynda's exquisite rendition of "One Hand, One Heart" from *West Side Story* — I clung to Geordie as if he were the only other person in the room. Our voices held as we said our vows, and we each remembered on which finger to place the other's ring. I smiled through our final kiss as trumpets heralded the recessional.

Besides Geordie's toast, which was a poignant, emotional tribute to his family and me that couldn't possibly be recreated in print, the highlight of our reception was the Anniversary Dance. All married couples started out dancing, and then gradually left the floor as anniversaries were announced. Obviously we were the first to leave. It was incredible to watch our parents up there dancing until 35, looking so happy with the other couples still dancing. Mom's friends, Willie and Dick Young, were the final couple, having been married for 42 years. It felt fitting to have the longest married and most newly married couples in the room both be Young's (although not from the same family) and I gave my bouquet to Willie as we posed for pictures.

After hours of dancing, cake cutting, and special visits with guests, the time came for us to leave. I couldn't believe it was over. It had absolutely been the most perfect day of my life, filled with more love and joy than I could have imagined possible.

The next evening, Mom came in to keep me company while I packed for our flight back to London, en route to Mauritius, for our honeymoon the next day. We smiled through our tears as we remembered the perfect day that had come from all our preparations. I had found and married my true love and best friend in a wedding that exceeded any expectations I could have had. Our conversation after

Drew's wedding, when we worried that she wouldn't be at mine, seemed so long ago. We had planned my wedding together, and had shared the whirlwind experience.

Mom and I cried through our airport goodbye, but I promised to call the next day before our flight from London — and that I'd see her soon.

INSPIRATION
November 2002 – January 2003

KAREN

Geordie and I had a blissful honeymoon of golf, snorkeling in the Indian Ocean, and relaxing by the pool in Mauritius. After ten days of indulgence, we were ready to return to our London routines, not to mention one course dinners. The sniper crisis ended with a double arrest on the 24th of October, to the relief of the Washington metro area.

I also returned to dozens of emails, including this special one from Mom.

Dear Karen,

The message attached is typical of the feedback I've been receiving. Although you set a high bar from save-the-dates through dinner favors, and including everything in between ... the really special aspects of the evening were your poise and radiance as well as Geordie's manner. It was a truly distinctive and memorable event for everyone who attended. Thank you so much for being my daughter and allowing me to participate.

Much love to you both.
Mom

Forwarded message from Claire:

… I'm wondering if you and Cliff have had a break yet. I feel privileged to have been invited to the wedding. It was so lovely. I saw you cry when Karen and her dad walked up the aisle. It was a touching moment among many. Several people wept when Lynda sang her song and Karen seemed genuinely to be moved by it. I would like to see Karen's train up close as Nancy and I were on the side in the pew…

The men at my table wept openly when Geordie spoke. I think you've got a good one there … Your silver dress was perfect. I hope you had a great time.

Karen must have talked to everyone at least twice, making everyone feel welcome and special. I'm happy for her.

See you soon, Vicki. Take care.

Love, Claire

I was concerned about the void Mom would feel after my wedding. It was clear that I needn't have worried. Soon after, she had the fall quilt retreat with Aunt Cyndi.

Plus, Neighbors Club, Garden Club, the Junior League Sustainers' group, and her Second Saturday Breakfast ladies each maintained their frequent activities. She had at least one fun activity each week.

Yet again, cancer also crept in to remind us of the reason she'd left work in the first place. Her CA-125 had been inching up for several months, but she'd firmly resisted commencing a new chemo treatment that would exhaust her. By early November it was 250. Her numbers weren't the only cancer frustration. November and December were filled with what seemed like excruciating doctor's visits for Mom.

Subject: Insomnia

Karen,

I'm so frustrated that I can't get in touch with you. I've been calling since before 3:00 A.M. (it's now 3:28 my time) and I keep getting the circuits busy signal. You must be in an early meeting.

… My day at chemo was less than fine. I was almost 10 minutes late, but waited an additional 35 minutes before I was treated … When I finally went back to the chemo room yesterday I sat in a guest chair — because all of the other five chairs were taken — during the first 45 minutes of my assigned appointment. Eventually, I was moved to a treatment chair.

Two of the nurses asked if anything was wrong because I was so quiet. I told them I was just tired. When one finally insisted, I told her about my long wait and the lack of communication between staff, since the nurses apparently didn't know I had arrived. I didn't address the lack of accommodations, although I did tell her I felt like a number rather than a patient.

… Actually I gave them a little tit-for-tat as I laid back and snored through most of the hour and a half I received the Doxil.

… Given my insomnia tonight — I've been awake since before two - I'm going to end this now (3:55) before I go back to bed and negate the possibility of your reaching me. Please call if you can; I'll keep my cell phone in my pocket so you won't wake Dad. Hope you're having a really good day!

Love you so much,
Mom

I was in meetings during Mom's insomnia, and read her email when I got back to my computer at noon — 7:00 A.M. her time. She was asleep when I called her back. A few days later, it was more of the same.

Subject: My appt

Karen, Lynda and Drew,

My CA-125 is elevated to 308 from 269 last month. My blood pressure was 160/110 but Dad thinks that might have been because I was shivering in the examination room and had waited over an hour and a half in the waiting room. I guess that would cause blood pressure to rise. My oncologist is taking me off Doxil and starting me tomorrow (unless the ice storm precludes my getting there) on Carboplatin, which is the first thing I had after surgery.

... I told Cyndi that I decided not to consult the cancer center oncologist about the change in protocol because I agree with my new doctor's rationale and am much more comfortable with her than I was with the first oncologist I had. I hope you concur. Consulting with the folks at the cancer center would delay the change in treatment at a time when my oncologist says the tumors are definitely growing.

... Sorry to relay such disappointing news, but that's all the news I have. The good part is that we're coming to London in a week and a half and to Mathews right after. I am so excited that I can hardly stand it.

Have a great day. Love you all so much!
Mom

Mom's escalating numbers threw me into a now familiar emotional tailspin. I wanted to DO SOMETHING, but I didn't know what. Every day I spent at Bain, working on an internal technology project that I found tedious and dull, I felt as though I should be doing something else. The difficulty was figuring out what that "something else" should be.

It came to me one night in early December, after lying in bed for over an hour with my mind racing. We needed to write a book about Mom's cancer. In the past, I'd always abandoned the book possibility for obvious reasons: I wasn't a writer; this wasn't about me; we weren't celebrities; and Mom had never shown any interest in writing about her cancer experience.

This time, the idea came to me differently. Maybe she AND I could write a book together.

The more I thought about it, the more I liked the idea. I'd never read the type of book I had in mind, in which two people tell the same story, each in her own voice. It would be similar to a novel in which each chapter is written from another character's perspective. But this wasn't a novel; this was a story about our lives. By incorporating my perspective as her daughter, the book would be differentiated from the myriad cancer survivor memoirs on the market.

As I sorted my thoughts lying in bed the following morning, I also realized that this could be a worthwhile project for us even if it were never published or read by anyone outside our family. Having a new project to work on together, as we had with my wedding, would give Mom a new goal to strive toward. At the very least, hopefully writing a memoir together would be a cathartic experience for us to share.

By the time the sun was rising over DC the next morning, I was so captivated by the idea that I was desperate to pursue it. Of course, Mom still didn't know anything about it. I was afraid that she'd immediately reject it as absurd, but I couldn't wait any longer to share it with her.

I suspect that I woke her up with my early call, but she said she was already up. I blurted, "I was awake most of the night thinking about an idea that I'm really excited about.

It's a bit crazy and you probably aren't interested for lots of reasons, but here it is." With that compelling sales pitch, I proceeded to tell her about my idea for our book.

She loved the idea! She said that she'd thought many times — throughout her life, and especially since her cancer diagnosis — about writing her memoir, but had always abandoned the idea as ludicrous. Her reasons for hesitating were similar to mine — she was just a "normal" person, and she wasn't a writer, so who would be interested? But, she was inspired by the idea of writing the book together — for many of the reasons that had led me to the idea in the first place.

She also raised the issue of her fatigue and questioned how likely it was that she'd have the energy to write diligently. I assured her that we'd take this at our own, relaxed pace. Clearly she then worried that I was going to backpedal our way out of getting this done at all, because she immediately insisted that we needed to set ourselves firm deadlines to make the book happen.

Within minutes of talking, we had committed to writing our story together, though a key question remained, which Mom finally voiced.

"Now that we're both committed, I have a question for you. Not to burst your bubble, but have you thought about how exactly you're going to fit this in?" Mom, ever the pragmatist, had realized that we'd talked about her time and energy for the project, but that I'd kept silent regarding my own constraints.

Realistically, I couldn't foresee writing the book while still working full-time at Bain. My first thought had been to ask for a six-month leave of absence to write, but that might pressure us to write more quickly than either Mom or I would be able to. Instead, I decided to ask Bain if I could work part-time while I wrote our book. As I hoped to be pregnant quite soon, I thought that my part-time could transition directly into maternity leave.

My Bain mentor was receptive to the project and sympathetic to the urgency to start while Mom was still able to write, but not to impose too much pressure by writing for six months full-time. We agreed that I would begin working 60% in January. Part-time is somewhat of a misnomer at a firm like Bain. The average Bain consultant in London works 55 hours a week, so my 60% schedule of at least 33 hours per week would bring me in line with the average full-time British worker.

My parents arrived just before Christmas to spend the holiday week with us in London.

Throughout the week, Dad watched numerous war documentaries on the UK History Channel as Mom and I began working on our book.

We decided to start at the beginning of her illness, and progress chronologically through to wherever we decided to end it. After a few hours of brainstorming, we had a rough outline that started a few months prior to her diagnosis and ended that Christmas. It became obvious to us that we should each write the complete story and piece our perspectives together, rather than trying to alternate chapters. Clearly, some sections would have more from her and some would have more from me, but we felt that this balance would be an important part of sharing each of our roles over the past few years.

Finally, we laid out some "Rules of the Road":

1. Have fun!
2. We're in this together.

3. We both write on each section and we'll piece it together in bunches as we go.
4. Karen will focus on the medical/research and any other yucky parts.
5. Afternoon Tea working sessions will be critical to success!

To get started on the right foot, Mom and I celebrated with our fourth London Afternoon Tea of the year — and decided that we could really get used to such regular treats!

My parents left on the 29th, to be back in time for Mom to resume Carboplatin on New Year's Eve Day. I finished the book outline while they were flying and emailed it to be in her inbox when she arrived at home. She replied that evening.

> Subject: Re: Chapter outline — just a few things to cover!
>
> This is amazing!!! I'll read it more thoroughly tonight or tomorrow and send you changes I think we need to make.
>
> Thanks again for a magical visit. We had a great time.
>
> Love you so much.
> Mom

Mom's first Carboplatin treatment in the third week of December had been an onerous experience. She had an allergic reaction to the treatment, and had to reduce the dosage several times over the course of the chemo session —

causing it to take much longer than expected for her to get the complete treatment. We hoped these difficulties would be a one-time occurrence.

She called on New Year's Eve Day, frustrated that her next session needed to be postponed because her platelet count was too low by five points — hers was 95 and the minimum for treatment was 100. She was asked to take Procrit and come back on January 2nd for chemo. To exacerbate her frustration, she arrived at the drugstore for the Procrit prescription only to learn that it had been left out on the counter instead of being refrigerated — so she needed to go to another store. Such glitches are annoying in everyday life, but can be intolerable for people with chronic illnesses like cancer, for whom the time and energy expended are truly precious.

Mom called me at work late on the 2nd. Her chemo session had been an unmitigated disaster, as her email later that night described.

Subject: Chemo session

Karen,

I'm writing this at around 7:45 P.M. on Thursday, and then going directly to bed. I want to send you the information before I forget the details.

... About an hour and a half into the chemo regimen, including premeds, I suddenly developed a severe reaction. I could hardly breathe, turned bright red, and began to sweat all over. All four nurses came right away and administered oxygen, a steroid, and Benadryl.

They also monitored my blood pressure and the level of oxygen in my blood and gave me cold compresses on my forehead and neck. It was really scary for about an hour.

I asked them to call Dad so he could come over and be with me, but they couldn't reach him on either his cell phone or office phone. This went on for almost two hours ... Then I asked them to call Cyndi. She came over and picked me up immediately, which turned out to be about 5:15. Dad insisted he was in his office but the phone didn't ring. Please discuss this with him, as he appears to me to be a little cavalier about my not being able to reach him. He implied that the nurses didn't really call him when I know that they did. It's scary that he isn't reachable.

... Because we are yet again between types of chemo, we probably should plan to connect with the cancer center oncologist and either talk with him or actually go to see him. We should set up a call to discuss.

Hope this hasn't caught you at a bad time. Have a good day.

Love you,
Mom

When Mom and Aunt Cyndi met with Mom's oncologist the following week, she was clear that Mom would be unable to continue on the Carboplatin regimen, even though her CA-125 had decreased by 100 after the December Carboplatin treatment. She recommended Gemzar, or gemcitabine, as an alternative treatment. Gemzar was primarily used to treat lung and pancreatic cancer, but she had seen some success using it as a second-line treatment for her ovarian cancer patients. Apparently, Gemzar has no cumulative toxicity, so Mom could be on it as long as it worked. And it wouldn't cause hair loss!

The doctor reassured Mom that if Gemzar weren't working after a few sessions, they could try a desensitization regimen of Carboplatin to try the drug again at a lower concentration, after pre-medications. This would make for a long, tedious treatment day, but was an option.

We all wanted to be sure that the cancer center team agreed with Gemzar as the next step. Mom's oncologist confirmed that she had been sending the consulting oncologist routine updates on Mom's treatments and diagnostics and was very amenable to including him in this decision point. I sent our consulting oncologist a detailed email on Mom's scores and treatments since her initial appointment with him a year earlier. I tried to call him late that afternoon, but he was in patient appointments. I waited as long as I could to leave the office for a work dinner; from the message he left on my voicemail, I must have missed his return call by only a minute or two.

I was awake half that night, frustrated yet again by the challenge of living across the pond from my family. I loved living in London — the verdant, spacious parks and architecture that ooze history and heritage, our wonderful cozy flat in South Kensington, and the opportunity for Geordie and me to start our life together in a new place. But I was made nearly insane by the frustration of trying to connect with friends, family, and physicians in the U.S., whose days started five to eight hours after mine.

It was the next afternoon before I finally connected with the cancer center oncologist. Fortunately, he agreed with all of Mom's local doctor's recommendations. Gemzar was considered to be one of the top three "second line chemotherapies" for ovarian cancer, along with Doxil and Topotecan, which she'd already had. If it didn't work, he also recommended the Carboplatin desensitization program.

January 9th was a better day.

Subject: Today 1/9

Dear Karen and Cyndi,

It's 8:35 and I'm being totally decadent. The best way to start the day is truly homemade English toasting bread with French quince confit. There's nothing better. The bed isn't made. My teeth aren't brushed. I haven't showered. But I thought I'd better sit down at the computer and write a little something so Karen doesn't finish the book without me.

The sun is out. The snow is melting. I just listened to a twenty minute oboe concerto on the radio and now have my favorite CD collection going in my office. What could top all of this?!

Have a great day.

Love you both,
Mom/Vicki

Later that day, Drew called me after he read my email about Mom's recent appointment. It was the first time we'd spoken in ages, and it was refreshing to hear his voice on the phone; from his email that afternoon, he felt the same way.

Subject: Hey sis

Hey Karen,

It was a really nice treat to get to talk to you today. It seems like it's almost impossible to keep in touch with our schedules, so it's nice to catch up whenever we can. I'm so happy for you that you are finally working somewhat "part time". I hope things work out so that you will actually be able to shorten your work week to some extent.

About these updates, I'm really glad you're sending them to me. I really like to know what's going on, even though I don't often reply to them.

… How's Geordie doing? Haven't heard much lately, but I'm sure he's doing fine. I just keep hoping that someday you all may decide that the Washington suburbs are the place for you (at least for a couple-year stint) so that we can hang out more. Anyway, really good luck on your book. I'm so glad you are doing that I can hardly put it into words. I can't wait to read it.

Love you,
Drew

Meanwhile, Mom's medical ordeal continued, as, miraculously, did her sense of humor.

Subject: Today's medical update

This morning I went for my blood test and the white cells were even lower than last week, so I won't be having chemo until at least Monday. I also still need Procrit for my red cells.

Tomorrow morning I need to go the hospital early to have a procedure referred to as "TPA" done for my medi-port. It takes four hours but I can show up and have whatever it is installed, and come back four hours later to have it removed.

Being a cancer patient is so much fun! One never knows how to plan actual fun activities because the medical appointments keep changing. The good news is that I should still be able to have my oncologist appointment when Karen is here next week.

Thanks to all for expressing so much interest in this ordeal. It makes it much more palatable.

Hope you are all having a great day. I'm going down for a nap now!!

Love you all so much.
Vicki/Mom/CA

After my first early morning writing rampage, I started to methodically write about the events of the last few years as we'd outlined. As it turned out, my "part-time" schedule at Bain ranged from 45–60 hours a week throughout January, which made it nearly impossible for me to find the time and emotional space I needed to collect my thoughts. Still, as I slowly completed each section, I sent it to Mom. She did the same, signing her emails "CA" for co-author. My mother far outpaced me in these early days of writing.

That Friday, I wrote my version of the chapter about Mom's first surgery. It was exhausting to revisit that week, but doing so refreshed my gratitude that she was still with us.

Subject: Re: surgery day

Wow!!!!!!!! Thank you so much for not sharing your notes with me until now. I'd had no idea of the surgical details.

… Don't ever tell me you don't have a great writing style!

Love you,
CA

I went to DC for a long weekend at the end of January, two days after my 30th birthday. I accompanied Mom to her regular oncologist visit that afternoon. Mom's new oncologist made me feel more confident in her capabilities each time I met her.

During our appointment, Mom asked her if she would be able to cure the cancer.

The doctor's quietly candid response was that it was unlikely. More likely, the cancer would stay as more of a chronic illness that can be treated. The goal was to keep it stable and controlled for as long as possible — like it was now.

Mom thanked her oncologist for being honest. When the doctor left the room, she looked at me and said, "I wanted someone else to hear that I'm not supposed to make it."

I was shocked. I didn't know what to say, so I put my arm around her shoulders, as she bit her lip to hold back the tears. I tried not to let her feel my body shake from the force of my own silent tears, which I couldn't hold back.

That night, I told my parents that Geordie and I were starting to try for a baby. Mom started to cry again, but these were happy tears.

"I never wanted to pressure you, but now that you've said that you're starting to try, I may as well tell you how much I really want to be a grandmother."

Dad and I smiled. She hadn't ever pressured Drew or me, but she'd talked about being excited to be a grandmother my entire life.

"So, do you think your sewing machine still remembers how to sew baby clothes, after doing so much quilting recently?"

"You'd better believe it does. I loved making clothes for you and Drew. You are going to have the best-dressed baby in London or the U.S. And actually," she started with a mischievous smile, "Liberty of London's lawn fabric is the best in the world for making smocked dresses."

"Why am I somehow not surprised that there would be a London shopping opportunity related to this news?" Dad countered in mock frustration. "Maybe I'll have to go to Holland and Holland [the premier custom gun maker in London] to have a gun refitted for the new arrival so I can take him or her hunting soon after its first steps."

I couldn't wait to have good news to share with them.

REFLECTIONS
February 2003

VICKI

Today I have lunch plans at Le Cote D'Or with Nancy. I try to limit my activities to one thing outside of the house each day unless I have errands to run — which I do today.

During my insomnia at three thirty this morning, I spoke with Karen and she said she was planning to write today — which I later learned she did, in fact, do. My routine these days is to devote mornings to the book and other household chores and sew in the afternoons. I'm so happy to finally have some sort of regular routine. It's easier this week because I have no medical appointments — very rare! Also rare is the fact that I'm not at all groggy. I'm only tired because I'm not sleeping well. It's a very good kind of tired, because it isn't caused by chemo or its effects.

Another significant change these days is my willing-ness to "wallow" in cancer and its issues. For the past three years I've been trying so hard to live a normal life, whatever that is. I wanted to keep my career, do a credible job for each of the kids' weddings, keep up the house, travel, and cook and sew on weekends as time permits. It just wasn't possible. With chemo impacting my schedule and how I felt, my already stretched schedule reached breaking point last March. Nevertheless, I still refused to become a "cancer patient" in my daily living. No group therapy for me. No other kinds of cancer activities. I continued to resist the thought of writing about my experience. I did, however, continue to read about other peoples' cancer and healing. But those books were worked into my reading schedule among novels and other nonfiction.

All that changed a couple of weeks ago. Karen and I started ordering additional memoirs and cancer resource books that might aid us in our writing process and I began to think about the cancer experience more and more. Just writing an hour or so every day kept it forefront in my mind. But the most notable change was when my friend Mary's husband Lou was diagnosed with colon cancer.

Although I resisted looking to others for help with my chemo and recovery process, I've discovered through Mary the need some people have to reach out. Now I spend quite a lot of time (relatively speaking, since I spend so little time on the phone with friends) talking to her about my experience and chemo in general. I've said all along that it's harder for the family and friends to cope with cancer than it is for the patient. Although it just isn't my style, I can help Lou best by being there for Mary. Hopefully I will remain an example of a person who is beating the disease and enjoying life to the fullest in the process.

It is important for me to have this message come through loud and clear in the book. It doesn't matter what color the ribbon, all cancer patients, and especially those undergoing chemo, have a common bond. I certainly didn't wish for cancer, but I'm quite happy that I'm able to be an example for others and be a support for their families and friends. I've begun to wear my teal ribbon with pride.

CO-AUTHORS
Spring 2003

KAREN

Geordie and I knew long before we were married that we wanted children — preferably as soon as possible, so my mother could meet and enjoy her grandkids. So, I met with an obstetrician for a "pre-pregnancy visit". He asked a few questions about my health and agreed to arrange some blood tests and an ultrasound scan to make sure there weren't any issues that could keep us from getting pregnant.

In early February, I found myself in an elegant private radiologist's office in a Victorian mansion flat in Marylebone. His antique desk consumed one corner of his office, in stark contrast to the modern examination table and ultrasound machine in the other corner. As I lay on the table, I thought ahead to the excitement of having Geordie with me looking at the ultrasound images of our baby to be.

The radiologist dictated his findings. "Uterus looks

normal … everything seems to be in the right place." Pause. "Ovaries are polycystic."

His pause and change in tone alarmed me. "What does it mean if my ovaries are polycystic?"

"Basically, it means that you aren't ovulating."

"Does that mean I can't get pregnant?"

"As long as your ovaries are polycystic, you won't ovulate at all, and therefore, won't become pregnant. However, polycystic ovaries are often treatable with hormones or surgical procedures." His response was matter-of-fact.

I was completely stunned as I thanked the doctor, left his office, and walked out into the light drizzle to hail a taxi. I called Geordie and asked him to come home early; I could tell he was worried, but I didn't want to talk about my appointment on the phone.

By the time I arrived home, I'd calmed down a bit by trying to focus on the doctor's assurance that treatments could help. I sat down at our laptop and Googled "polycystic ovaries". I immediately wished I hadn't. The websites and articles that came up about polycystic ovaries, and polycystic ovarian syndrome, varied from mildly reassuring to dismally depressing. I learned that it was thought to be the leading cause of infertility among otherwise healthy women of childbearing age.

I had hoped to wait to call Mom until I had enough information not to alarm her. Instead, I called her newly upset from what I'd read.

"Hi, Mom, do you have a few minutes?"

"For you, I have all the time in the world. Actually, I was just finishing some writing, so your timing is impeccable. How was your day?"

"Well, I went to my ultrasound appointment as part of

my pre-pregnancy exam." I tried to just relay the facts, but was already crying again. "Oh Mom, it looks like there's something wrong with my ovaries." I described my appointment, and the information I'd read online.

"It was so awful to go to what I thought would be a routine exam, and instead find out that I have a medical condition I've never heard of that might keep me from having children. I can't even imagine how it was for you in all of your early appointments, being alone when you found out you had cancer. I've thought about it before, but it never hit home like it did today. I'm so sorry you had to be alone for all of that."

"Oh honey, it was terrible, and I wish you hadn't had to endure a similar experience. But, it's all over now and the only thing to do is to move on. Have you talked to Geordie about it yet?"

"Not really. All he knows is that the appointment didn't go well, but I didn't want to give him the details on the phone."

Just then, I heard Geordie's key in our door. Mom and I said good bye quickly, and I promised to call the next day.

Geordie walked over to the sofa where I was sitting and moved me onto his lap. I put my arms around him and just sobbed for a few minutes while he held me. He was comfortingly reassuring and proactive after I shared what I'd learned.

"You know we're going to get through this, don't you? It isn't great to hear that there might be a problem, but at least we know about it now and can work on fixing it as soon as possible. This is the whole reason we decided to get tested up front, isn't it?"

It didn't make me feel much better, but he was right. Three weeks later, we met again with the obstetrician, who tried to keep us from being alarmed by the ultrasound. He thought that my body could just be taking time to regulate after going off the pill and encouraged us to wait at least six months before exploring fertility treatment options. I appreciated his non-alarmist attitude, but I was also unwilling to just wait and see, so started to do fertility research on my writing days.

From her emails, it seemed that Mom had similar plans:

Dear Karen,

That last chapter was wonderful and I cried through most of it, even though I had read lots of it before. You are really a very expressive writer. I promise to get some writing done on Saturday. Now I'm off to Web MD to find out what I can about polycystic ovaries.

Love you so much, my first-born who made me a mother!!
Mom

One day, I didn't feel like writing so instead I plotted her CA-125 test results into an Excel graph as a tool for writing the book. Her original score of 1200 didn't even fit on the graphs (if it did, the scale would cause the other scores would disappear into the x-axis). I sent it to Mom and family as a bit of perspective of the roller coaster ride it had been, and the current trend.

Dear Karen,

Thank you so much for doing this. It's a great experience to do projects with an MBA. Even if you are at home for the rest of your life, don't ever try to convince me that Stanford wasn't worth every penny — and not just for the Geordie experience.

Keep up your spirits. If I can lick cancer, you can conceive a child.

Have a great day.

Love you so much,
CA

I smiled when I got Mom's email. She had a rare gift for making me feel better.

Amidst her pep-talks, Mom was writing up a storm, embracing her new co-author "CA" status. I spent the rest of February trying to get as much written as possible so she and I could edit and compile our work when we were together in March.

It wasn't easy. Looking back, I realized that I'd been a self-centered jerk for much of the period of Mom's diagnosis. Worse, writing about her early appointments and surgery brought back heavy feelings of dread and uncertainty. I couldn't imagine how it was for Mom to relive these experiences, but she was writing too, in between treatments and dealing with everyday life.

Ah, the last chapter you sent was much more entertaining and less of an emotional experience. It's now eight in the morning here and I'm off to shower, dress, et cetera. I'll be home all day except for a brief sojourn to the grocery store. Call any time if you wish.

Love you,
CA

The first week of March, I had a business trip to New York that I was able to combine with a visit to my parents in DC. This time, Mom came with me to one of my doctor's appointments, instead of the other way around. The fertility expert referred by her friend was incredibly helpful by email even before our first appointment. His style was refreshingly American, as he described the implications of PCOS (polycystic ovarian syndrome) and discussed treatment options that he'd recommend for someone with my patient profile.

In a role reversal from our typical appointments, Mom helped me answer his questions about my health and family history. I hadn't remembered having amenorrhea in high school, but apparently this wasn't a new problem for me. We also discussed the new potential family risk of ovarian cancer, and he said that he would take this into account when considering hormone treatments. Like my doctor in London, he encouraged me to wait six months, but at least gave me a sense of what our next steps would be.

There was no such wait for my mother, who had taken new ownership of her own medical journey, as evidenced by her update emails.

Subject: Latest Update

My apologies for being so tardy in getting this update to you. Dad asked me to send it out on Friday and I got completely caught up in other things.

My oncologist appointment went pretty well, with both good news and bad news. The good news is that two of my tumors are continuing to shrink. The bad news is that the other one is growing and my CA-125 doubled to 224.

This was only my second cycle on Gemzar so I will have one more (3-week) round of it — starting tomorrow. After that I will have another CA-125, mammogram, chest x-ray, and MRI; then will see my oncologist again prior to going to the cancer center again in April. After the trip, the doctors will decide on the best course of action. I continue to be anemic and Dad is still giving me my weekly Procrit shots.

Just remember, it could be worse. We'll keep you updated. Have a great day!!

Love you all,
Mom

A few weeks later, Mom came to London for a "writing workshop" weekend. We'd each written several chapters of the book at this point, so this was to be the first test of how it would all fit together.

Subject: Book files

I'm sending you each file separately as I'm not sure AOL is savvy enough to include more than one attachment in an email. I'll log on once more before I leave today. If you don't receive any of these, let me know and I'll send again.

See you so soon.

Love,
Mom (CA and chief visitor to Onslow Square)

Mom arrived on a Thursday when I was at Bain. She rested from her flight and was refreshed when I got home that evening. By the time Geordie arrived, we'd devised our strategy for tackling the book that weekend.

We had a marathon editing day on Friday, including intense reading and a lot of patting each other on the back. This was working! Of course we were incredibly biased, but we were each really pleased with how it was turning out as we combined five chapters of our separate writing into one cohesive story. We didn't agree on everything, but we did on most sections and on others we took turns deferring to each other. My only concern was making sure that Mom shared enough of her side of the story. In contrast, I tended to share too much, veering wildly off-topic.

By Saturday morning, we were desperate to get out of our small flat! We decided to take our work into the garden. One of the best parts of our home was the private garden square, just across the road. Geordie and I hardly ever used it, but we often saw children playing or adults picnicking on the lawn. The gardens were immaculately maintained in controlled clusters of flowering shrubs, trees, and fields of daffodils that were in perfect bloom that early March.

Over the course of the weekend, we spent several hours on one of the garden benches, handwriting new material. Sometimes, I found that writing by hand helped me write more freely than I could facing a screen. Not this time — I was distracted by Mom's presence next to me and found myself just soaking in the chance to be with her in the gorgeous garden. We talked more than we wrote and the rest of the weekend flew by, aided of course by Afternoon Tea at Claridge's Hotel.

Mom left Monday morning and was back on email that night with details of her cancer center preparation.

Subject: Films

On Friday, March 28, I am having my MRI at 8:00 and my chest x-ray and mammogram later that morning. I will have my oncologist appointment here the following Thursday and will send the films to the cancer center by Fed Ex overnight so my consulting oncologist will surely have them by my appointment on the 15th. I'm sure the films will not be academy award quality but they'll be the best I can muster.

Love you,
Mom

_____

Subject: our trip

Your chapter 7 is wonderful!! I especially like the paragraph with the plea for apheresis donations. It is truly part of the healthcare process.

Also, I booked our flights today. The tickets were expensive, but there's nothing we can do about it. We'll just have to make every minute of the trip count — writing, editing, resting, shopping, visiting quilt shops, et cetera. Maybe a little sightseeing if there is anything of interest ...

Love you so much.
Mom (CA)

Amidst our planning for the cancer center visit, I forwarded her some information I got from the Ovarian Cancer National Alliance about possible publishing resources for our book. I smiled at her reply.

These are great ideas. By the way, you know how Dad and I do so much in odd years (like getting married, buying our first house, and having our children). I have great vibes that we are going to not only write but publish the book in 2003!

Have a great day and thanks for calling earlier.

Love you so much.
Mom

Mom had a gift for keeping my spirits up, especially on my more challenging writing days.

Dear CA,

I think the only way writing will get easier is to do more of it. Practice not only makes perfect, it makes it routine.

I hope to get some writing done this afternoon before I need to go to the blood test. I still haven't had lunch yet, so that's next.

More later. Love you.
Mom

_____

Dear Karen,

See attached very short chapter 9. I will augment later. I never did get to the chapter about Drew's wedding, but will work on it on Sunday as time permits.

Love you so much. See you on Monday afternoon. I hope the trip won't be too taxing for you. It's almost as far as my trip with your dad from DC to Africa!

CA

Because my "part-time" case schedule in January had comprised 45-60 hour weeks, I was able to accompany

Mom to the cancer center without taking holiday time. It wasn't the ideal premise for our annual mother-daughter trip, but under the circumstances, it would do.

As grateful as I was that Dad and Aunt Cyndi had accompanied Mom on her first visit to the cancer center, I was excited that this trip would just be the two of us. My Aunt Cyndi had recently decided to leave her career as a business communicator in order to pursue her dream of starting *Moonlighting Quilts*, a multi-faceted art quilting company. Her ulterior motive, which she downplayed to Mom, was to have more flexibility and time for her sister's health. It was an amazing sacrifice for her to leave her successful career to follow her heart, and she was in the final stages of this transition during our week at the cancer center. Dad stayed home to work, and to give us some mother-daughter time.

Just as Aunt Cyndi had done the prior year, I sent a thorough email recap to the family to let them know what we found. My email was typical of the update emails that she, Dad, Aunt Cyndi, or I were sending at least monthly at this point.

Subject: Mom's appointment update

Dear all,

Well, it's nearly noon in London, so I guess it's about time I'm up and writing just after five in the morning local time! First, I want to echo the positive impressions of the cancer center that Mom, Dad, and Aunt Cyndi had last year. This place is extraordinary. I'm typing this in a 24-hour resource center with nine Internet-enabled computers and a library of books for guests to read at their leisure — just one indication of the way they cater to guests and patients.

… Based on Mom's test results and our meeting with him, the consulting oncologist recommends that Mom try Carboplatin again (the one she reacted to at the end of December) administered with a desensitization protocol, so hopefully she'll get the therapy's benefit without an adverse reaction … A likely scenario would be course one next week, course two after San Francisco, before London, and course three after Paris. It even fits her luxury travel schedule!

After the Carboplatin, there are other chemotherapy options, plus clinical trials … Most trials are administered by subcutaneous injections, and the trials run by this cancer center could likely be administered remotely, maybe even by Dr. Greve in the granite procedure room (translation: by Dad in their kitchen).

The oncologist characterized Mom's cancer as "not curable, but not terminal". This means that she still responds to treatments and is in a very stable condition.

So, that's the scoop! I hope you all have a wonderful day. I'm off to run on the treadmill, and then I am donating platelets this morning. After that's done, we're writing! We would be shopping, but we cleaned out the Galleria Mall last night …

Love you all,
me

After sending my email, Mom and I traipsed all over the hospital looking for the apheresis center, where we talked for two hours while I donated platelets. We devoted the afternoon to the book and talking about our lives in general. We combined a few more chapters, and revised the outline to include the past few months. We joked that this book might never end if we just kept adding chapters.

Mom had already thought of this and had a solution: "We'll stop the book when there are no big things looming; when everything is stable and life is happy."

This worked with her new life philosophy that she was trying to follow. "I'm trying to be totally selfish for the first time in my life; not self-centered, but self-oriented; doing what's right for me."

What was right for her on Thursday was a drive to a quilt store in a seaside town about an hour away from the cancer center. Mom bought many yards of fabrics in her post quilt retreat enthusiasm. We also each bought some teal colored fabrics, as Aunt Cyndi had been encouraging us to do given that the teal ribbon is the symbol for ovarian cancer.

We had a casual seafood dinner early that evening overlooking the water. Even in mid-April, it was beastly hot on the restaurant's deck, without any semblance of a breeze on the waterfront. As we fanned our faces with our menus to cool ourselves while waiting for our drinks, Mom and I shared our gratitude for the chance to be together while gaining reassurance about her treatment options.

Mom had another appointment with her local oncologist the Tuesday after returning from the cancer center. Dad sent out the update that afternoon.

Subject: Mom's oncologist visit

The doctor feels that the vaginal tumor is a little larger. She seemed a little reluctant to go with the revised Carboplatin protocol, but agreed to do it ... It has to occur on a day when the nurses aren't too busy, and when she is in the office in case of a reaction. She promised that it wouldn't conflict with Mom's travel schedule coming up.

Mom asked the oncologist whether the disease was worse. She said that it wasn't worse, in the sense that there probably wasn't more disease, but that it had advanced a little in that it had developed more resistance to drugs. She said that, even if it responded to a particular chemo and virtually disappeared, it would probably not be cured since it would be very likely to come back ...

Basically, pretty similar to what the cancer center oncologist said.

Love, Dad

Two days later, Mom was back in her oncologist's office after a night of severe vaginal bleeding. She was also starting to have more pain in that area. The doctor on call thought the bleeding was probably caused by the vaginal tumor and triggered by Mom's two internal examinations within two weeks. We all felt the urgency to begin effective treatment immediately, and Mom had her first Carboplatin desensitization treatment a week later.

Subject: chemo

… Tomorrow, I have to leave the house at 6:45 A.M. Ugh! That's the time when Dad generally brings me my first cup of coffee. I need to be there at 7:15, which is the earliest any of the nurses will be able to begin my chemo. Nobody knows how long it will take. I'm hoping all day, since that is the plan unless I have a reaction again. I'm really hopeful that it will work out this time.

Have a great day … Thanks for all the writing, etc. Love you so much.
CA

She had very minor reactions, but was able to complete the treatment session. I edited the nine chapters we'd worked on together on our trip and sent them to her. I sent additional chapters to Mom as I wrote them, which wasn't as often as I wanted it to be. Her responses cheered me on.

Subject: Hello CA! Here's chapter 11

What a powerful chapter. I really loved it! You are such a good writer; I'm not sure why I'm participating in authorship.

… I'll be home all day except for groceries and a noon manicure/pedicure. Have a great day!!

Love you so much.
Mom

Of course, Mom's medical ordeal continued.

Subject: today's appointment

Hi all,

This morning Dad accompanied me to my regular oncologist checkup. It was a very good appointment with positive results except for the CA-125 which went up from 358 to 398. The doctor was not concerned about the rise as it wasn't very great and she said we can't expect a lot of progress after only one round of Carboplatin. My second round is tomorrow.

… Although my red and white cells are in the normal range she wants me to continue with Procrit and Neulasta (at $2,500 per shot!) because she thinks they are responsible for my improved blood counts. The other good news is that the tumors are not growing and in fact one seems to be shrinking. Yeah.

On a lighter note, I had a fabulous surprise yesterday. Periodically at quilting meetings there are quilts offered for raffle. I won a queen-size quilt that won second place at the November quilt show in Houston in the category of quilts made by groups. The quilt top was machine pieced and hand appliquéd by the Old Dominion Appliqué Society. The best part is that the colors are perfect for Drew's old room. I can hardly wait for you to see it. It's truly magnificent and I really love it.

Have a great day all.

Love you,
Mom, Vicki, CA

Despite Mom's upbeat email, she was in significant pain, and she was constantly tired. I could tell the difference on the phone with her each day. She sounded exhausted and dejected. She still tried to stay upbeat, but it was clearly a real effort to do so.

Aunt Cyndi's next post-chemo update email began:

To quote Vicki, "Well, for the third day in a row I saw my oncologist." Yesterday, Vicki's body went into anaphylactic shock and decided that it didn't want any more Carboplatin. So, today we went to talk to her doctor about what to do next.

Her oncologist presented five chemotherapy regimens she could do, or she could participate in clinical trials. She promised to expedite the process for Mom to be seen, so that her treatment could resume as quickly as possible. The only decision now was which treatment to pursue.

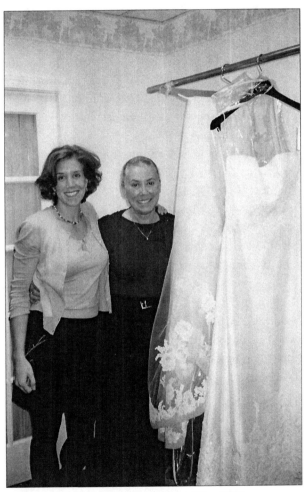

Karen and Vicki at Karen's first wedding gown fitting, 2002

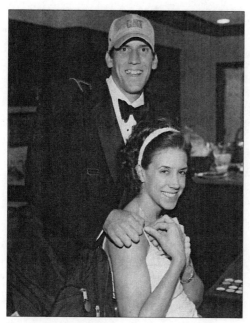

Drew and Karen the morning of Karen and Geordie's wedding, 2002

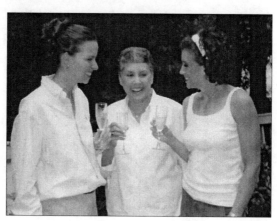

Anne-Marie, Vicki and Karen enjoy a celebratory pre-wedding toast

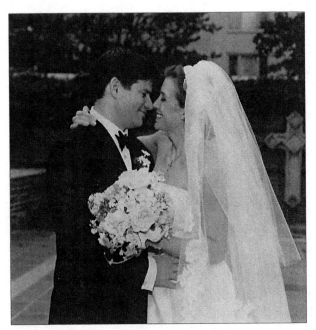

Geordie and Karen share a wedding day moment, 2002

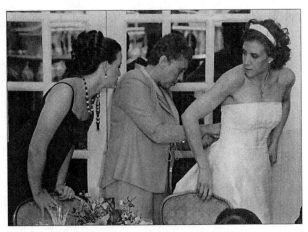

Anne-Marie and Vicki fix Karen's bustle ... again, 2002

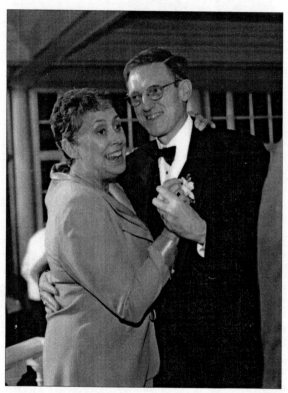

Vicki and Cliff during the Anniversary Dance

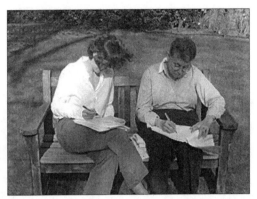

Karen and Vicki writing in the Onslow Square Garden, 2003

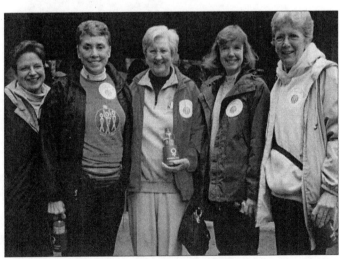

Second Saturday Ladies Carole, Vicki, Jean, Willie and Nancy at the Virginia Walk for the Whisper, 2003

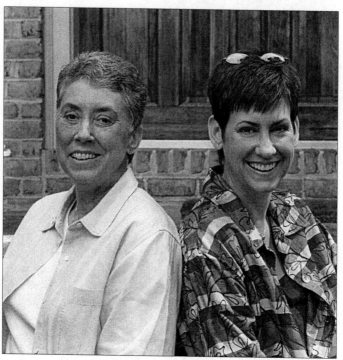

Vicki and Cyndi enjoy sister time, 2003

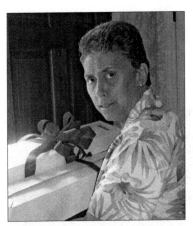

Vicki receives three dozen roses from Cliff on their 36ᵗʰ anniversary, 2003

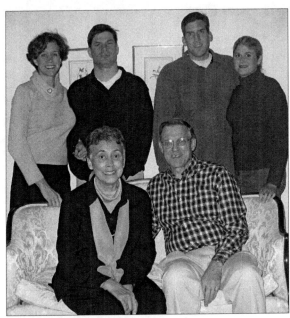

Karen, Geordie, Vicki, Cliff, Drew and Lynda, Thanksgiving 2003

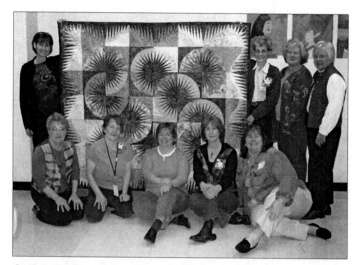

Cyndi (back, left) and fellow quilters with Teal Beauty, 2007

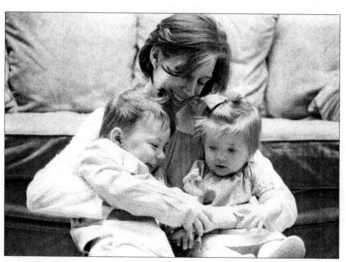

Jeffrey (3 ½), Karen and Kathryn (10 months) during their last month in London, 2008

TRAVELS
May – June 2003

KAREN

One evening in May, I received a call from the Nominating Director of the Junior League of London (JLL). She was calling to ask if I'd be the Community Research Director for the year starting in June. I agreed to speak with Beth Franklin, the current Community Research Director and soon to be Community Vice President. I didn't know Beth well, having only met her at the two Community Research meetings I'd attended since joining the JLL in January. My initial impression was that she was a bright, passionate woman with a bit of an artistic flightiness. I had been shocked to hear that she had teenaged kids; she was a slim blonde woman who looked just a few years older than me.

I called Beth, certain I'd decline the position. However, I discovered on the phone that Beth is a master of persuasion. She convinced me that the Community Research Director role provided a relatively easy entrée to a charity Board of

Directors position, without much additional work beyond the monthly JLL Board meeting.

Geordie wasn't convinced. "You already talk about being stressed out and overwhelmed. Have you thought about how you are going to do this on top of everything else? Obviously, it's your decision. But something is going to have to give at some point."

"I know, but I think this is a unique opportunity to get into the charity sector at the Board level. Besides, I don't think it will be too much work if I set my boundaries."

Geordie raised his eyebrow and smirked at me. "You realize that you won't set boundaries; you don't know how to do anything half-way. I'll try not to say "I told you so" when it gets to be too much."

Mom was totally supportive. In her Junior League, which she served for many years, including as President, Community Research Director was a big deal.

"I think you should be honored to be asked and embrace the opportunity. I never regretted the roles I took in the JLNV [Junior League of Northern Virginia]. I enjoyed every one and they were a huge influence on my career."

"But, this might cut into my time for the book. I haven't been the most productive writer recently even without this new commitment."

"Don't worry. We just need to arrange some more motivating authors' trips. My visit in a few weeks will get us back on track. Speaking of which, have you decided where we're going to take the ladies to tea?" Our conversation digressed to her upcoming visit to London with the Second Saturday ladies and other plans for the summer.

With Geordie's support and Mom's encouragement, I accepted the position. In the next two days, I received a deluge of emails about the upcoming Board Retreat and transition meetings. Maybe this was more than I'd bargained for. I'd soon see.

In June, Mom arrived for a visit with three of the other Second Saturday Ladies: Nancy, Jean, and Willie. The four of them had been friends for decades; three of them were past Presidents of the Junior League of Northern Virginia. The ladies stayed at an updated traditional bed and breakfast around the corner from our flat, and mostly did their own activities — sightseeing, visiting Kew Gardens, going to West End shows, and shopping. They came over one evening for dinner at our flat and, of course, we went to Afternoon Tea.

Each time I saw her, Mom radiated enjoyment and exhaustion. The ladies were careful to limit walking and activity, but they were all energetic, fit women just as Mom had been before her cancer, and I could tell that even their moderate pace was a stretch for her. They saw it too. Nancy and Jean each took me aside at points during their visit to share their concern that Mom was overtiring herself. She insisted to them, and to me when I asked, that she was "just fine."

It wasn't until after they left on Sunday that she confessed to me that she was completely enervated. "Would you mind if I took just a little nippy nap in your guest room? We can talk about the book in a little while; I just need to rest first." When I woke her for dinner, she couldn't believe that she'd been asleep for over five hours.

"I probably shouldn't have pushed myself so hard with the ladies. They were so sweet, and kept asking me if I needed to take more breaks. Of course I did! But I didn't want to hold them back or miss out on any of the fun. I'm so tired of being the cancer patient. It seems like everything exhausts me these days. Will you please help me take it a bit easier in Belgium and France?"

The "real" purpose of my mother's visit was to attend the wedding of our French friend, Elé. She had been a close family friend ever since my French teacher arranged for us to be pen pals when I was in the fifth grade. Mom and I adored her, and Mom was determined to go to Elé's wedding, no matter how she felt.

On Wednesday, we flew to Belgium to visit Victoria for two days en route to France. Mom loved lace and delft pottery, two reasons why I was especially keen for her to visit Belgium while Victoria was still there doing research for her PhD. Mom tried to act captivated by the charm of Antwerp, the university town where Victoria and her fiancé, Robert, lived. But she was still tired from London and had trouble walking on the cobblestone streets. After a quick tour of the cathedral, we had an early dinner so she could rest.

We slept in as late as we possibly could before our train to Bruges with Victoria the next day. In Bruges, Mom's breathing was really labored as we walked around the shops, but her face beamed as she looked at the lace.

After much searching, we found the perfect tablecloth for my dining room table. It combined the intricate, web-like lace that I preferred with the eyelet accents that Mom favored. Unfortunately, it was staggeringly expensive relative to some of the others in the shop.

Mom hadn't noticed yet. "This is just exquisite. Look at the intricacy of the handwork. It's one of the most special tablecloths I've ever seen. But don't get it just because I like it. It's for you, so you need to love it."

"Oh Mom, did you look at the price? It's much too dear. I don't know when I'll ever have a special enough occasion to use it — and would probably be afraid to! I can see the red wine stains now. Let's keep looking."

"Are you finished?" Mom cocked her eyebrow and gave me her characteristic "I'll humor you by listening, but we're doing this my way" look. "This is the nicest and largest shop we've seen and that tablecloth is perfect — we even both like it. I don't care how much it costs; I want you to get something you'll always treasure."

With that, Mom handed it to the shop merchant. Victoria had observed our exchange with amusement. "Now I know where Karen gets her stubborn generosity with gifts. It's fun to see her be the person who doesn't get to say no, for a change."

Mom left the shop with new energy from her purchases, but her pace slowed again after a few minutes. We stopped at a café to rest and enjoy an early lunch.

"Well ladies, Bruges is lovely, just as promised and I've had my lace fix. Shall we head back to Antwerp?"

"We can, but don't you want to look at the delft pottery before we go?"

Mom smiled. "Not me, I just spent my travel budget on your tablecloth! Just kidding. But, I don't need any pottery, and if we bought some we'd have to carry it for the rest of the trip. Let's just head back after lunch. You girls would probably enjoy some time by yourselves, and I wouldn't mind a little nap."

Back in Antwerp, Victoria and I went for a walk. She confessed that she was surprised by how much weaker my mother seemed than just eight months earlier at my wedding.

"I know, and the really scary thing is that she's making a huge effort to rally during our visit."

We continued along the Antwerp waterfront, talking

about Mom, Robert, my fertility issues, Victoria's research, Geordie ... skipping from topic to topic. I wished she lived in London.

Back in the hotel room, I waited until the latest possible minute to wake Mom for dinner. I sat on the edge of the bed and put my hand on her shoulder. "Mom, did you have a good nap? It's time to get ready for dinner."

Her eyes opened slightly. "Already? I feel like I just fell asleep." She'd slept for four hours.

Dinner was amazing, at one of the best restaurants in Antwerp. I couldn't understand how the French maintained the title of best cuisine in the world, when Belgian food was similar, but a bit lighter and without the haughty attitude.

The next morning, we had an errand to do before our train to Paris. Mom's oncologist and the chemo nurses had endorsed her prolonged holiday only on the condition that she have a blood test midway to be sure that her blood levels were stable. This was only the second time she'd been away from home for more than six days since her diagnosis nearly four years ago.

The hotel receptionist directed us to a doctor's clinic, just a block away. In the pristine, well decorated clinic, Mom chatted with the doctor while he put on his gloves and took her blood. In perfect English, he confirmed the tests he'd process on her blood samples and promised to send the results to Mom's oncologist's office. Two hours later, we were on the train to France.

Later that same day, we arrived at Les Chandelles, a tiny village near Chartres. Our quaint five bedroom inn was one of ten ancient stone buildings in the village. Soon after arriving, we were sitting on wrought iron chairs in the back yard surrounded by lovely gardens.

"To our mother and daughter vacations," Mom toasted, as we sipped the Kir Royales that had been offered by the proprietor. We could definitely get used to this.

It was beastly the next afternoon when we arrived at La Mairie (the Mayor's) for Elé's civil wedding ceremony. Afterwards, we were supposed to proceed by foot, along with the rest of the guests, through the ancient town of Auffargis from La Mairie to the church. But between the stifling heat and the hilly route, we decided to follow in our rental car instead, watching the colorful parade of wedding guests that could have been a scene in a period film. The reception was at a gorgeous chateau with cocktails outside and dinner indoors. Throughout, Elé and her parents treated us as family, introducing us to the other guests as part of her father's welcome and including us in some of the family pictures.

I started to worry about Mom as it became clear just how long French wedding receptions were. The six courses at dinner were punctuated by a magician circulating among the tables and lively dancing. At two o'clock in the morning, *la bouche* (wedding cake) was presented and I finally felt that we could excuse ourselves. We were the first to leave! I couldn't even imagine how tired Mom must have been, but she raved about the wedding until she left for home the next day.

Mom's visit in June marked the beginning of a summer in which Geordie and I only had a few weekends in London without house guests. I knew I should feel lucky that we had so many close friends and family members coming, but it had reached absurd levels. Not only were we going to be inundated by guests, but they all planned their visits to include the weekends on either side of their trips. I felt suffocated by the prospect of only a few weekends at home with Geordie. To exacerbate the issue, my home office did double duty as our guest room, so I had to work around our visitors' schedules. I felt as though I'd lost my summer before it had even started.

That wasn't the worst of it. Dad was furious with me for how ragged Mom was when she returned home to DC. He conceded that he knew the trip was special for her, but he was really worried about her. It was the first time he'd audibly voiced his concern about her health in a long while. In addition to her extreme fatigue, she'd had increased vaginal bleeding and problems going to the bathroom. Her CA-125 taken in Belgium was up to 547.

RADIATION
Summer 2003

VICKI

My oncologist's recommendation, coupled with the wisdom of the consulting oncologist, was to seek the help of a nearby research center that was running a clinical trial for ovarian cancer. My oncologist referred to it as a "third opinion". My tumors were growing, and more were appearing, according to the three big indicators — my CA-125, MRI, and physical examination. All of the most attractive chemo regimens had been tried and I had either used them to the max (Taxol), or was allergic (platinum based drugs, like Carboplatin), or they hadn't seemed very effective. I was ready to try anything, so I agreed to participate in the clinical trial.

However, before I could begin the clinical trial protocol, I had to undergo radiation on the large vaginal tumor that had been bleeding intermittently, sometimes excessively. The doctor leading the clinical trial explained that, should bleeding occur during the trial, I could be required to end my participation. Thus, I faced a delay while I sought radiation treatment.

My oncologist recommended a renowned local radiation oncologist. I liked her instantly, as well as the rest of the radiation team. They took photographs of my face as well as the area that was to be treated. I was also measured from every possible angle to ensure that the radiation would affect only those cells that needed it. For some unexplained reason, the measuring process took over an hour on a very hard table. I could hardly wait to get off of it, and sincerely hoped that the staff's assurance that the actual treatments were short was, in fact, accurate. All of the team members were quite knowledgeable about every aspect of the treatment and I was truly pleased to be in such good hands. The downside was that I would see this staff of experts every weekday for the next six weeks.

Each new cancer treatment has brought its own surprises. Radiation was no different. I had no shortage of friends, relatives, and medical folks who told me what to expect. The big three were sore skin, diarrhea, and fatigue. Since sore skin and fatigue have plagued me since the first chemo session, I thought I was prepared for them. Diarrhea was a different matter. In truth, I had been dealing with constipation for more than three and a half years and was looking forward to getting that out of my life. The nurses gave me powder for my skin and medication for diarrhea.

While the side effects weren't expected to show up until about the third week, fatigue was a factor instantly. My days became a routine of showing up at radiation by 9:15 A.M., having treatment, going home, and napping. The whole radiation exercise took about an hour and a half every morning, including travel time, wait time, and less than fifteen minutes on the table. I'd been given a special parking permit for radiation patients, and parking was free, so at least that part of the commute was painless. I drove myself for the first four weeks, and Cyndi or Karen drove me for the final ten sessions. At that point, I could hardly get out of bed in the morning, much less drive twenty minutes to the hospital by myself.

The radiation oncologist had said in passing that radiation should buy me a year. Did that mean I had a year to live, or that I'd now have an extra year? It seemed to me that people were treating me differently now. Even my therapist was so sympathetic that I began to dwell on just how sick I really was. In addition, since I'd had no chemo or other treatment since May, and it was now July, the cancer had been having quite a growth spurt. I could feel the tumors getting larger, and my CA-125 test results just kept getting higher and higher.

A side effect I didn't expect was depression. I realized that radiation was a "last resort" treatment for me, since it could only be administered once on any given part of the body. The clinical trial was also a last resort for me, in that I had already been treated with all of my best traditional options.

Instead of thinking about a better future without the tumors, I dwelled on the fact that I probably wouldn't live to see my grandchildren. Although both of my children were now married, grandchildren were probably still a few years down the road.

I began to avoid going places, seeing friends, even talking to my children on the telephone, which I used to enjoy so much. I had liked working on the jigsaw puzzle in the radiation waiting room, so I got out one at home. I frequently couldn't even muster enough interest to do something as mindless as that. Bills went unpaid, and more and more duties around the house were falling on Cliff's shoulders. I just continued to get more and more miserable. It didn't help that we were having an extremely rainy spring and summer.

Food tasted terrible to me, and I completely lost my appetite. In all I lost about eight pounds during radiation — not a lot for a dieter over a six week period, but I had been admonished not to diet. My weight was supposed to remain stable.

I have a wonderful sewing room full of projects that I'd been looking forward to doing, but I no longer even wanted to go into the room. Karen and I had started to write this book months ago, but I just couldn't bear to sit at the computer and write anything during this period. The subject was loathsome to me, and weren't such books generally written by survivors? I didn't expect to survive much longer.

DECISIONS
July 2003

KAREN

Mom called one evening just as Geordie and I were finishing dinner.

"Hi sweetie, I'm just about to take a nap but wanted to call first to see if you got Dad's email." Mom's voice was so low on the phone, that I had trouble hearing her.

"Not yet. Is everything OK?"

"It's just as well that you haven't read his email; it isn't very cheerful. I'm not OK. I haven't been OK in so long that I don't remember what it feels like. It hurts so much down there, and the bleeding is getting worse. I'm afraid to even leave home for long because I need to be near a bathroom to avoid accidents. This is the pits." Her voice broke as she spoke. She hadn't sounded this depressed in a long time.

"Oh Mom, I'm so sorry. Hopefully the radiation will start to make it better soon."

"I know; I'm sorry for calling. I hate complaining and I feel like it's all I do these days. I'm going to go to sleep now and maybe I'll be in a better mood when I wake up. Have a good night."

"Are you sure, Mom? I'm here if you want to talk more."

"No, what I probably need is sleep. I'm just so tired. Enjoy your evening and we can talk tomorrow. I love you"

"Bye, Mom. I love you, too."

After we hung up, I opened Dad's email. Mom's CA-125 was over 900. I tossed in bed that night, worrying about our conversation and realizing that I needed to be with Mom much more frequently than I could manage with my current commitments.

My new case at Bain had very manageable hours, but bored me to frustration. On my non-Bain days, I juggled Junior League calls, emails and meetings, managing our flat, fertility appointments, brief attempts to write the book and as many conversations with Mom as she could handle and I could find time for. Each time I voiced my feelings of being overwhelmed, Geordie's predictable reply was, "You're doing too much. You need to cut something out."

With Mom's latest results, I finally knew what had to go: my job at Bain. I got up early the next morning to figure the financial ramifications of losing my salary — which we could just manage.

I shared my thoughts with Geordie as soon as he woke up.

"I know that this will have a massive impact on our finances, and that I'll be away from you much more than I want to be. But Mom needs me, and I don't have much time left with her."

Geordie's reply was immediate and supportive.

"I'm really proud of you and I think this is the right decision. Don't worry about money. If we can't get by on my income, we have even more problems than these. I'll miss you when you're in DC, but I'm not going anywhere and you need to do what's right for you and our family."

That night, Geordie and I talked more about the logistics of my quitting on our finances, family planning, and my travel away from him. Then, I called Mom.

"Are you sure?"

It was at least the fifth time Mom had said these three words since I'd told her about my decision to leave Bain.

"Completely. Are you sure it's OK for me to come home for several weeks in July and August?"

"Oh, Karen." Tears almost quelled her voice. "It's always OK for you to come home. You know that. I feel like I shouldn't let you do this for me, but I'll be so grateful to have you here more."

"Then it's settled. And I'm doing it for many reasons. You're the most important, but it will also enable me to focus on my charity interests and giving you a grandchild."

"Actually, that's the most important reason of all! But have you stopped to consider how you'll get pregnant when you're here and Geordie's there?"

I had, and it was going to be a challenge, although I didn't divulge this to her. I'd created a calendar on graph paper of the next few months. Diagonal lines going in one direction indicated days when Geordie and I would be together, but not in London where my fertility clinic was. Crossing diagonal lines showed days when we would be apart. There were very few clear days in between for the remainder of July through September. I didn't share with Mom that we were probably going to take a couple of months away from trying for a baby until then.

The next day was Tuesday July 1st — Canada Day and Drew's birthday. My shoulders felt lighter with my Bain decision made, especially since it was a non-Bain day. That afternoon, I attended my first Junior League Board meeting. I was energized by the dynamic in the Board Room, where former and practicing lawyers, consultants, investment bankers, and other professionals strategized how to take the League forward in the coming year. As a new member, I felt intimidated at first, but by the end of the meeting I was comfortable expressing my opinion on the issues at hand — as I usually am.

On Wednesday, I scheduled a meeting with my Bain mentor. While I waited to see him, I opened my email to see that our cancer center oncologist had responded to my update on Mom's condition and new CA-125 score:

Subject: Re: Victoria Greve medical status

Hi Karen

I am sorry to hear about the status of your mother. Unfortunately, this is a terrible disease and her condition will hopefully improve with the proposed treatment. However, I think we should be preparing for the fact that as time goes on she may continue to deteriorate without us being able to help. This will be a very difficult time, but I will certainly help you and her with everything I can.

Stay in touch,
P.

I gasped for breath as my tears blurred the message on the screen. I'd known ever since it had become apparent that Mom's cancer wouldn't recede into true remission that eventually we would be forced to face the reality of losing her. Reading the doctor's message on my screen brought the reality crashing home.

I was almost late for the meeting. My mentor suggested that I take a Leave of Absence, rather than resigning in a time of personal crisis. I thanked him for his kindness, and Bain's ongoing compassionate support of my situation.

After my meeting, I received an email from Mom responding to my email update to her cancer center oncologist. I hadn't shared his reply with her.

Subject: Re: Victoria Greve medical status

Thanks for doing this. Today is a really yucky day — both dismal skies and personally poor attitude. It could be related to not getting much sleep last night and overdoing it in my closet cleaning exercise. Aunt Carolyn is coming for lunch, so I know that will perk me up. Did I share the wonderful email she sent the other day? I'll send it separately. She's also offered to help take me to appointments.

Have a great day.

Love you,
Mom

Karen,

Isn't Carolyn's message nice? See below.

Dear Vicki,

Thank you for the update on you. It is easier to write the details than to tell them repeatedly. I wish the news was better, and I am so sorry that you are now having pain. I know that sounds hollow, but there is no other way to say it.

I won't say this to you again, so you don't have to worry about me getting mushy when we are together. You have shown such depth of character and courage throughout all of your pain and illness. You have made it easy for people to be with you, and I am proud to be your sister-in-law and friend. Plus, you have given a wonderful legacy to your kids about how to handle it when life dishes out its evil. They will always have the example of your grace and caring for others instead of yourself. They will also know that the only thing we can really control is how we deal with what life dishes out, and you have dealt with this in a truly magnificent manner.

I know that I have only seen your public face, and that you must have moments of great despair and sadness, but the fact that you have held it together publicly is remarkable. So now I have said what has been in my heart. You can be proud of yourself, my Boomer!

Carolyn

Aunt Carolyn is my father's sister. She and Mom had been roommates and best friends in college, which was how my parents met. I was glad she and Mom were reconnecting, but it was a small solace that day.

When Geordie got home from work that night, he sat down on the sofa and I crawled into his lap, sobbing. When I could finally speak, I told him about Mom's most recent test score and the oncologist's email. At least I no longer had any lingering doubt about my decision to leave Bain.

Geordie and I attempted our first round of fertility drugs that July: five days of the lowest possible dose of Clomid, followed by a series of ultrasound scans to track the progress of my ovarian response. Nothing happened. Every scan showed that my ovaries were still polycystic.

Conversations with Mom were less consistent.

One day she was particularly upset after her doctor's appointment, during which her doctor used terms like "rapidly growing tumor". In a dejected voice, she told me about the rest of the day.

"Cyndi and I went to an antique store after my appointment and I saw a painting that I really liked. But then I thought that it would just be another thing for Dad to have to get rid of. It wasn't the sort of art he particularly likes and it isn't fair to saddle him with it."

The next day, she was like a different woman entirely.

"I'm going to lick this, I just am. I feel achy and painful, but not sick."

"Wow, you sound much better."

"I am. I refuse to let this get me down. You heard it here first … this cancer will not get me!"

A day later, we spoke for nearly an hour. It was longest conversation we'd had in weeks. Then suddenly, I heard a loud crash and she abruptly ended our call. I phoned back several times before she finally answered. She confessed that she'd fallen down and felt so humiliated that she hung up the phone.

"I'm a little hurt but mostly just really embarrassed. I scraped skin off my right knee and left elbow. How did I manage that?"

"You must be my mother. I don't know anyone else uncoordinated enough to manage such a feat."

"You'd better watch out or I'll get you back for that comment! You'll be here soon, you know."

"Less than a week. I can hardly wait."

"Me too. Now, my knee really is throbbing. I'm going to lie down, but don't worry about me. I love you."

"I love you too. Keep that leg up. Bye Mom."

My last day at Bain was Wednesday, July 23rd. The next evening, Geordie and I left for New Hampshire for Victoria and Robert's wedding. It was the first time that all eight of my Harvard roommates had been together since Hilary and Stephen's wedding in April 2002. With our partners, we comprised a third of the fifty guests at the wedding.

As Victoria's "best woman", I accompanied her to her hair appointment and helped with her makeup and dress, giving me precious time alone with her on her wedding day. We should have spent the entire time talking about her wedding, but I also gratefully accepted her advice and support as I prepared to go home to my parents that Monday.

When Mom had told me that the radiation oncologist thought the radiation should "buy her a year", my first response was elation. After reading the oncologist's email, which I never shared with her, I didn't expect Mom to survive until Christmas, much less an entire year. For Mom, I think it was the first time that she started to absorb how little time she might have left.

Ever since Mom had resigned her body to surgery and chemotherapy, she'd compensated with emotional courage and character that sustained her alongside the rest of us. She'd certainly had moments in which she'd openly shared her feelings of frustration with the cancer that threatened to rob not only her dignity and energy, but also her life. But these were compensated by her fierce will to survive every indignity and pain with style and grace. In the tension between determination and desperation, determination had always prevailed — at least before radiation.

The day after I arrived in Virginia, it took much, much longer for me to rouse Mom from bed and help her get dressed than I'd anticipated. By the time we pulled into the parking lot for radiation, we were running terribly late. She directed me to the "Radiotherapy Patients Only" parking spots just outside two glass doors.

"Nice, Mom, we got the last one. These are even a step up from the handicapped parking sticker."

"They should be. People just don't understand how awful radiation is. It's hard enough just to get here, much less to walk any further than necessary."

We got out of the car, and I was surprised when she walked in the opposite direction of the glass doors.

"Mom, where are you going? Isn't this our entrance?"

"I'm checking to make sure that all of these cars have the proper radiation tags. See," she gestured to a midsized silver sedan, "this one doesn't have the tag."

"Maybe they just forgot. Besides, there isn't anything we can do besides be grateful that there was still a space left for you." I heard my mother's typically rational, understanding words coming from my mouth.

"Oh yes, there is. It just makes me so angry."

After a short walk that was still arduous and painful for Mom, we finally arrived at the radiation wing. She alerted the receptionist that there was a silver sedan illegally parked in the radiation spaces. I had the impression from the receptionist's response that it wasn't the first time this had happened. It was the first time I had ever seen Mom lash out in such a vindictive way against an anonymous offender. It felt like she had started to hate her life.

When I called Aunt Cyndi that evening, I wondered if I was being melodramatic.

"Karen, I'm sorry you had to see that, but you're right. It wasn't the first time. This radiation has been the worst thing Vicki's endured. It's been a month already and can't be finished too soon. She's just exhausted. I know it might not make you feel better, but your visit really has helped to lift your mom's spirits."

"She was worse before?" I just couldn't believe it.

"Let's just say that she's really happy to have you home. I know it's a hardship for Geordie to have you gone, but it's a lifeline for her to have you here as much as you possibly can be."

"Thank you. I think it's harder on me being away than on Geordie, but it really helps to know that it makes a difference to her having me here. Sometimes I feel like I make things harder instead of easier."

"Believe me, you make things better. It's the cancer that makes everything harder than it ever should be."

It got even harder the next day. Ten minutes into Mom's appointment with her therapist, Carter opened the waiting room door and asked me to join them. I had taken Mom to many of her appointments with Carter, and this had never happened. Mom was crying in her chair when I came in.

"I asked Carter to get you; you deserve to hear this too." Her voice broke and she blew her nose before continuing. "I'm so sorry to have to share this with you. I told Carter that I was dreading my next CA-125 result, so she suggested that I call from here." Her pitch increased as she blurted, "It's 1265. That's even higher than when I was first diagnosed!"

I put my arm around her shoulders.

"I'm so sorry Mom."

I was stunned and nearly speechless. I felt I was encroaching on their private session, even though I'd been invited, so after a few minutes I returned to the waiting room.

I tried to take a few notes for our book, but I was incapacitated by the dread of finishing the story without Mom, a recurring horror that had overwhelmed my writing efforts all summer.

OCCASIONS
August – September 2003

KAREN

On Friday, I flew to Toronto to meet Geordie and drive to Restoule. I had only been home for five days, which felt both much too brief and yet like an eternity.

Vivian was sitting outside the cottage when our car pulled in; I wondered if she'd been there all day eagerly waiting. This trip was the first time that I shared our fertility struggles with the Youngs. Geordie told me that he didn't mind my telling them, but he didn't want to do so himself. I think it was sometimes harder for him to talk about it than for me, since all of our issues related to my body. One morning while Geordie was still sleeping, I told his parents. I'd dealt with the situation for so long, that I was surprised when I had to suppress tears while divulging it to them. I almost broke down completely when Vivian reassured me that there was no rush, and that everything would work itself out in due time. I shook my head until I was able to find the words, "I know, but for my mom there isn't time."

As usual, Mom and Dad picked me up at the airport when I flew back a week later. Radiation was finally over and Mom mentioned several times how happy she was to be done with "that awful ordeal."

On my second morning in Arlington, I heard my parents go downstairs and stayed in bed, my knees still covered by the quilt Mom had won at the auction. I couldn't miss this opportunity to capture my parents' morning routine and scrawled longhand on a pad perched on my knees:

Each morning of my stay, I hear Dad's footsteps descending the stairs to start breakfast at six thirty. He pours water to fill the Mr. Coffee, then measures two rounded scoops of Maxwell House into the filter. While the coffee brews, he carefully counts out Mom's pills for the day. They come in all shapes and sizes and have a tendency to get lost in the flowered placemats she made. By now, the coffee's finished brewing and I hear him quietly creeping upstairs with two full mugs of coffee, and then softly open the door of their bedroom.

A few minutes later, he is dressed for work and has gone back downstairs to finish making breakfast. He calls up to Mom, "Breakfast, honey." It's the second or third time he's called her, and this time she stirs. She pushes back the covers and slowly gets out of bed. She pulls down her bathrobe from her dressing room and picks up her now tepid coffee to begin her protracted walk downstairs to breakfast.

Mom eats slowly and deliberately. She's scarcely half finished with her sliced peach when he eats the last bite of his breakfast. They talk about the day ahead. He gets up to do a few things around the kitchen while she finishes eating. This used to drive her crazy, but now she's resigned herself to his need to stay active and is grateful that he continues the conversation while she eats. When she's eaten all she wants — never her entire breakfast these days — he clears all the dishes and puts them in the dishwasher. With a kiss, he's on his way to work.

This unvarying routine adds an hour to my father's day. It wakes my mother several hours before she needs to be up for her first appointment. More days than not, her next two hours are spent napping on the family room sofa, just four feet from the breakfast table.

Family breakfast has been a daily Greve ritual for my entire life. As a young child, I took it for granted. As a teenager, I resented its intrusion on my time and flexibility. I can only imagine the deafening quiet at the table when Drew and I left for college. When we came home for school holidays, it felt as though we'd never left.

Now, the table dynamic feels different. My parents have moved beyond us, in the best possible way. They still clearly love us and cherish the time that we're all together, but they've found each other again and have reclaimed their places foremost in each other's lives.

When Dad used to kiss Mom goodbye and tell her each morning that he loved her, it seemed more like a habitual recitation than like an expression of feeling. Sometime in the decade since Drew and I left, that changed. Nearly forty years into their relationship, my parents are more in love than I've ever seen them. Dad now spontaneously looks at Mom with a glint in his eye and takes her hand in his. Now when he tells her he loves her — more often than at his daily departure and arrival home — his voice is rich with emotion and caring.

After her post-breakfast nap on Tuesday morning, August 12th, we went for Mom's blood test, and stopped for ice cream at Georgetown's famous old fashioned ice cream parlor en route to her appointment at Carter's. Mom's appetite had waned to such an extent that part of my role was bribing her to eat — with an emphasis on calories. She joked that her butter pecan ice cream cone was her favorite treatment yet.

By the time we returned from our morning adventures, Mom was ready for a nap. She was on her way upstairs when the doorbell rang.

"Karen, do you mind getting the door?"

I opened the door, and called for her. "Mom, it's someone for you."

"Who is it? I'm not expecting anyone."

"It's a delivery for you. I don't think I can sign for it."

She sighed. "I'm sure you can, but that's OK. I'll be right there."

Mom was flabbergasted as the delivery person handed her an oblong white box, then a second one and finally a third. I offered to carry them to the kitchen while she signed for them.

She counted as she opened the boxes.

"Three dozen red roses? Is your father crazy?"

"I don't think so. After all, you have been married for 36 years today. Which is just incredible, by the way."

Mom had told me many times how for their first few anniversaries, he'd given her the same number of roses as the number of years they'd been married. After about six years, he'd started to give her an even dozen; she joked it was because he could see that their marriage was going to last and that their anniversary was going to become very expensive. She'd always said that she was going to ask for fifty roses for their golden anniversary.

She had clearly been thinking of the same story and her face suddenly clouded over as her eyes filled with tears.

"You put him up to this, didn't you? Is this because you don't think I'm going to be here for our 50th Anniversary?"

I was crying too.

"He did it because he just loves you so much. He wants every year to be special."

"But I don't have many left. I'm not going to be here next year. You know that, don't you, and so does your father."

"Oh, Mom. No one knows how long you'll be here, but you deserve to enjoy every special day you can. Three dozen is a lot of years! You deserve to celebrate."

She gave me a tired smile and surveyed the expanse of roses waiting to be arranged. Normally, she couldn't wait to start trimming ends and placing flowers in vases; this time I could see that the prospect was daunting to her.

"How about if I arrange them and you can either supervise or fix my mistakes later?" I offered.

"Oh, if you would do them, that would be wonderful. I'm sure you'll do a fine job. I never thought the day would come that I wouldn't want to arrange flowers, but I'm just not up to it." She paused. "I'm going to go take a nap. I love you."

She kissed me on the cheek before turning to shuffle upstairs.

Mom's Second Saturday breakfast moved to the third Saturday that month, and Dad and I picked her up directly from the restaurant to drive to Mathews for Lynda's show at Donk's. I'd never seen Lynda perform her own show, rather than supporting a cast performance or singing in church. No wonder Drew had fallen in love with her the first time he

LOVE YOU SO MUCH

saw her at this very show three years earlier. She electrified the stage, keeping the sold-out audience enraptured through both acts. Mom slept both ways on the drive so she could rally her energy for our visit with Drew and Lynda.

At our appointment the next day, the oncologist provided a clue to Mom's exhaustion. Her blood work had revealed that her red blood count was at a precipitously low level. Mom's doctor was shocked that the radiation team hadn't prescribed Procrit for her and wondered aloud whether this explained most or all of Mom's fatigue. The rest of the appointment was somewhat encouraging, as her tumors seemed to have gotten smaller, though her vaginal tumor was very painful during the exam and her CA-125 had nearly doubled, to 2143.

I boarded my flight to London that evening hoping that the Procrit would magically revitalize her before my next visit in a month, and that Mom's pain from radiation would finally dissipate. She tried so hard to focus on the positive, and on everyone else, but she was really struggling.

Subject: My day — Wednesday

My dearest Karen,

Please don't share this email widely because it is too private although a lot of folks already know what I'm writing below. I hope it isn't too hard on you for me to lean on you this much.

It's late and Dad is in bed. As soon as I lay down I started to cry — I've done a lot of that lately. This was such a difficult day and I need to start putting some of this stuff in writing before I forget just how hard it is. I really hope you don't mind my sharing it with you. Hopefully you can help be my memory when we get to this part of the book.

A friend called to invite me to lunch tomorrow because she'll be in town for the day. I turned her down because I'm just too tired and know I won't have the stamina. I felt terrible about doing it but think it was the right thing.

While Cyndi was here at noon I really cut her short when she started giving me advice about how to better organize the sewing room. I just started to cry and told her I had a hard time getting up in the morning and getting dressed. I don't want ANY advice about how to organize the house or the rest of my day. I hope I wasn't too harsh with her but we had a similar conversation yesterday about medical advice. Won't she ever understand that I want companionship, but not any advice or suggestions of any kind?

That's all I seem to get from everybody. All the well people I know have all the answers about what activity will make me feel better when I'm so anemic I'm border line for needing a blood transfusion and can barely get through the day ...

In the mail I got a get well card and four page letter from a fellow quilter — from whom I never usually hear except in group missives for the entire eight of our retreat committee.

When I was on the phone this afternoon, another friend dropped off a package with a coping with cancer video and companion book and a note that I haven't had the courage yet to read.

Then Claire called (we never communicate except group emails and the Second Saturday gatherings) to ask how I'm doing. She's a pediatrician and wants the full skinny in medical terms. She always says don't talk about it if you don't want to, but continues to ask anyway.

This might sound crazy, but all this caring is making me so sad. All I want is to feel better and live to see my grandchildren — I truly don't think either one is in the cards for me. In the meantime I'm trying to live as normally as possible with a deepening depression and flagging energy. I'm at wits end and my nerves are really on edge.

The best part of my life is Dad. He really knows how to deal with me and when to step in and when to back off. I don't know how he became so sensitive when the rest of the world is totally missing the picture. You and Drew are also exceptions. I'd really like to hear a little more often from Drew, but, because that wouldn't really be our natural pattern, it's OK with me for now.

I'm planning to try to have a good cry and get some of this out of my system so I can sleep. My schedule for Thursday is to get up with Dad — and stay up! I have a manicure at 3:00 P.M. My only other plans are to pay bills and hopefully do some ironing with my wonderful new iron.

I'm so sorry to be sharing such heavy stuff with you when you're the daughter and should be the one leaning on me. Feel free to call when you get a chance. Hopefully I'll be feeling better by then.

I love you so much.
Mom

Mom was mostly down these days, as her email reflected. I felt guilty all over again for being away from her, even though I knew I needed the break — such that it was. I had two days in London with Geordie before Anne-Marie and J arrived.

Subject: visitors

I had no idea you have only one day between visitors. No wonder you are trying so hard to get things done. Only you could handle it well and still make your guests feel welcome.

Have a great day.

Love you so much,
Mom

Just after Anne-Marie and J's fun whirlwind visit, the Youngs came for a five week visit to England, Scotland, and France, using our flat as a base. Although part of me longed for down time alone with Geordie, it was comforting to have them, especially Vivian, staying with us.

I'd often worried that Geordie's parents were skeptical of my decision to stop working at Bain in favor of staying home. I hoped that seeing me flit from meeting to meeting, coping with the dozens of charity-related emails I received each day, and speaking to Mom several times daily would help them to realize that I was still doing worthwhile endeavors — not just aimlessly wasting my days. I knew they would have supported me regardless, but it was important to me that they see me as a meaningful contributor to our family.

When they'd planned their visit, I hadn't anticipated that I'd be gone for nearly a third of it. Two weeks after they arrived, I left for the Ovarian Cancer National Alliance Conference in San Francisco. I had business cards made in anticipation of this trip, on which I followed Mom's advice to use my full name, "Karen Greve Young." She was finally starting to sound more energetic now that she was a couple of weeks past her radiation ordeal.

Subject: Can't sleep

It's almost eleven at night and I've been home from the quilt meeting for well over an hour. Since I really can't sleep, am in great pain in the back and side, and am starving, I decided to get up and have a snack of yogurt and write emails until the sleeping pill takes over.

Today was truly one of the busiest ones I've had in a long while. I did errands and saw my psychiatrist this morning. Then had a sandwich for lunch and saw Carter at two. After that, I made brownies for Dad, I went to Fairfax to pick up a jacket and pants I had on order, stopped at a deli to buy another sandwich for dinner, and went to Cyndi's to go to the quilt meeting with her. Hopefully I'll begin to have similarly busy days more often ...

Have a great day.

Love you so much,
Mom

All looked positive going into her clinical trial protocol. Her CA-125 was stable, albeit hovering staggeringly high at around 2200. The only new symptom was that she was seeing an odd halo effect out of her eyes, which the doctors planned to check out before she started the clinical trial protocol.

I was almost at the front of the queue to register for the ovarian cancer conference when my cell phone rang.

"Hello."

"Karen?"

Mom's voice had the forced cheery but almost tinny tone that meant that she wasn't doing well.

"Hi, Mom, I'm literally about to register. Can I call you back in five?" As soon as I asked this, I remembered that her clinical trial had started today and reconsidered. "Wait, no, let's talk now and I'll register in a few minutes."

"No, you go register now and call me back. I'm afraid you'll be upset after I tell you why I called."

I registered in a fog, collected my conference materials and found a quiet place to call her back.

"Hi Mom, I love you." I didn't know what to say, or what had happened, and on the phone I felt helpless to do anything but give her emotional support.

"I love you too. I'm so sorry to call with a bad update. Again. Do you want the punch line?"

"What happened?"

"Today has been a wretched, awful day. I saw an eye doctor at the research center that's conducting the clinical trial. He said that I have glaucoma in my right eye." Her voice started to break. "And I have cancer in my left eye."

"Oh Mom. Is Dad with you?"

"No, he's helping Drew move back into his house and deal with the trees uprooted by Hurricane Isabel, which is the most important place for him to be right now. Cyndi's here with me, and has promised to stay with me all day. I don't know what I'd do without her. When they first told me about … the cancer in my eye, I screamed and said, "Oh no, it's too awful." I couldn't help it. I think I'm still in shock, but it helps having Cyndi here and talking to you."

"Oh Mom, I wish I were there with you too. Do you want me to come home?"

"I have to admit that I thought about it. But no, I want you to stay at the conference and get ideas and contacts for our book. Maybe you can also ask if anyone has had a similar experience of cancer spreading to their eye, and what they did."

"Of course I can, if you're sure. Are you OK to tell me about what the doctors said, or do you want to talk more later?"

"I don't think I can, but why don't I let Cyndi tell you? She's been taking copious notes, as always, and will give you a better idea of the next steps. Here she is."

I waited for Mom to pass the phone to her sister. "Hi, thank you so much for being there with her. I don't know what any of us would do without you. How is she?"

"She was pretty rattled, understandably, but is doing better now." Aunt Cyndi relayed the sobering details to me. Mom would have eye biopsies today, and would be disqualified from the clinical trials protocol unless her eye was cleared. The doctors said that it is exceedingly rare for cancer to spread to the eye and were considering her options. She'd probably be on radiation for a few weeks.

"I hate to ask, since you've already done so much, but can you take her to her appointments until I get home in a few days? I can come home early, and stay longer, if I need to."

She responded quietly, so Mom wouldn't hear. "You do what you need to do there. I'm fine with her — remember that she's my sister and is as much my responsibility as she is yours. This sort of thing is exactly why I stopped working, and I'm here to help her in any way I can."

My Aunt Cyndi was amazing that entire week, as she had been for months before, and Mom shared her gratitude in an email.

Subject: Thank you

Dear Cyndi,

Thank you so much for doing this update and for giving me your entire day and evening yesterday. You are so much more valuable and important to me than you could ever imagine.

Cliff is sending a separate email to everyone with comments about today's visit to radiology. The gist as I remember it:

- If we don't do radiation, I risk detached retina or worse
- Sometimes the radiation itself causes blindness
- When I asked about the urgency of radiation, he said it should start on Friday instead of waiting until Monday. I was thinking more in terms of weeks, not days.

What this all brings home to me is that I need to change my focus. In addition to the letters I want to write (which I had better start sooner rather than later) and the book I am co-writing with Karen, I need to see to my office, sewing room, and closets. While I'd love to come and watch you sew and do my needlework there, I think I need to spend the bulk of my time at home getting my affairs in order. This is so hard for me, but at least I have a chance to do it.

Thanks so much for your continued support. We'll talk soon.

Love you,
Vicki

Admonished to stay at the conference, I tried to absorb as much information as I could from the lecturers and other attendees. It was an extraordinary group of people, mostly women survivors — or "thrivers" as they called them-selves, as most continued to live with cancer — and medical professionals, with a few family members and friends also attending. Others' stories alternately made me feel lucky for the time we'd already had with Mom and afraid of what was ahead.

I spoke to Mom each day during breaks between sessions. After one of these conversations in which she described the awful mask she wore to clamp her head to the table for the radiation, I practically ran to the nearest ladies room, where I sobbed uncontrollably in the privacy of one of the stalls. I struggled for ten minutes to regain enough composure to rejoin the conference. I splashed cold water on my face, but still had red and puffy eyes when I went back to the lecture. I had the impression that I wasn't the only attendee whose emotions overcame them at some point during the week. Many of us were united not only by our commitment to improving diagnosis and treatment options for ovarian cancer patients, but also by the ravaging impact of the cancer on our own lives.

On Friday night, I took a red eye flight to spend the next week with my parents. Each morning that week, Mom had daily radiation treatments, in which they clamped her head into the special mask on the cold, metal table to keep her perfectly still for the treatment. The doctors didn't know whether the radiation would restore the vision in her left eye — and wouldn't know for several weeks. All we could really do was cross our fingers and pray.

At least her oncologist confirmed that Mom's tumors were all much smaller at her next appointment. The vaginal lesion that had caused so much bleeding in early summer was almost gone. So at least the horrible radiation ordeal of the summer had shrunk Mom's largest tumors. But, Mom no longer qualified for the clinical trial because of her eye tumor.

Mom's oncologist started the conversation about next steps by asking Mom's thoughts. Mom replied, "What are you going to give me to start beating this cancer?"

The doctor's face broke into a smile and her response was, "If you said you didn't want to do anything, I'd try to talk you out of it. There are still several things we can do and I feel positive that we can fight the cancer back. We're going to try to outsmart it." She outlined a plan for using Topotecan chemotherapy weekly to maximize results with minimal side effects.

One afternoon, Mom went with me to see the fertility doctor in DC. I asked if she wanted to rest instead of coming, but she quipped, "It's about time that I go to a doctor's appointment for someone else; everyone keeps coming to mine."

The doctor validated the fertility plan that my London clinic had already recommended for me to pursue as soon as I was able to return to London for a sustained period of time. Now, I just needed to get back to London.

CELEBRATION
October – November 2003

KAREN

Mom finished her eye radiation on the first of October, a day before originally scheduled, after subsequent tests revealed that her eye problem wasn't cancer at all. It was a virus that was so rare that the eye specialists only saw about one case a year, almost always related to severe immune system problems like AIDS or transplant anti-rejection medication. They suspected that hers was caused by her long bouts of chemotherapy.

She was lucky that she hadn't gone blind in her left eye while she was subjected to nearly two weeks of unnecessary and high risk radiation. Not to mention that the incorrect diagnosis disqualified her for the clinical trial. Now, she needed to start antiviral eye drops immediately to kill the virus, and then have laser surgery to repair her retina.

Dad's latest email update documented an array of appointments, but at least the prognosis was improving. In two days, she'd been to one hospital for her eye, seen her internist, and had her regular oncologist appointment. It appeared that the virus in Mom's eye was finally healing, and she could start to phase out her various medications. Her internist was concerned about the pain in her side, and thought that it could be metastasis of the cancer into her rib cage. Her oncologist agreed to order an MRI to be sure, but thought this was unlikely. The CA-125 result hadn't come back, but the doctor felt that all of Mom's tumors were smaller from the continuing effects of the radiation that summer. She recommended postponing chemotherapy until Mom was finished with her eye medications, and would see her in a few weeks to plan the next treatment protocol.

Overall, that was what passed as good news these days. It lasted three days. After several tries on Monday, I finally reached Mom at Aunt Cyndi's.

"Hi there, how are you doing?"

"I don't think you want to know." Uh-oh. "My CA-125 has doubled. It's almost 4000. Cyndi was with me when I found out and we came over here to play with fabric and distract me."

I couldn't believe it. How high could it go? "Mom, I don't know what to say. I'm so sorry I'm not there with you."

"It wouldn't be any lower if you were here, and to be honest, I don't know if I believe the number anyway. I don't *feel* like my CA-125 has doubled, so I'm going to pretend it hasn't. What I really want to hear about is your anniversary weekend in Scotland."

I told her all about our weekend golf trip at Turnberry, one of the British Open courses. As I described the scenic vistas on the course, playing up the Scottish brogue of my caddy and elaborately recounting our delicious meals, I was distracted by her CA-125 score, "almost 4000."

It amazed all of us how well Mom seemed to be doing, despite her high CA-125 and manic appointment schedule. She seemed to be on a mission to spend more time on fun than on medical matters — which was quite a lofty goal given her myriad weekly appointments.

She didn't yet realize it, but her optimism was supported by hopeful happenings in London. After seeing how depressed and dispirited Mom had been on my last visit, I decided that the best thing I could give her was a grandchild to look forward to. I started a five day cycle of Clomid hormones on October 8th, just before our first anniversary. It was a relief to have begun the process — and I tried not to obsess about the implications of the little pills I took each morning.

Ten days later, my ultrasound scans finally looked different. One of my follicles was growing! We were finally at the "trying" stage, and were instructed to "try" the next night, and following morning and that evening.

I felt like I was walking on eggshells for those next two weeks. Mom and I talked even more than usual, thanks to her new energy level. My challenge was to keep from divulging the status of our pregnancy efforts to her. I was desperate to tell her, but afraid to disappoint her if this cycle didn't work out.

Her emotions and thoughts seemed like a yo-yo. Generally, she was much more upbeat than she had been in months, but I sometimes feared that she was trying to pull the wool over our eyes and hers. She had always been such a vibrant, energetic woman, and was clinging to this identity even when she felt awful. Her social life at 58 made mine at 30 look absolutely pathetic. That Saturday night, Geordie and I were having two couples over for a low-key dinner. Meanwhile, she and Dad had not one, but two parties — a black tie gala for the Arlington Free Clinic, of which Nancy was Executive Director and Mom served as a Board member, and Aunt Cyndi and Eric's annual Halloween party. I wasn't too surprised to see Mom's email the next morning.

Subject: Oh, I feel terrible...

Dear Karen,

It's 1:15 A.M. and I'm still up — or rather up again. We got home from Cyndi's party just before midnight and were in bed within twenty minutes. I just couldn't sleep. My side was throbbing and my stomach was making weird noises just like every other night. When I'm up and doing something, my mind is occupied and I don't notice the pain and upset stomach as much. But bedtime is something I've come to dread. Dad made me a cup of tea before going back to bed, and also gave me a Percocet and Ativan. Together they should knock me out, but it hasn't happened yet.

The Clinic Gala was really quite nice. The theme was "A Thousand Points of Light" to celebrate the fact that this year they were a recognized charity by the Thousand Points of Light Foundation...

We saw so many friends whom I only see at functions like that. Everybody said I looked so good and I was laughing with the best of them. If they only knew the agony I'm experiencing whenever I sit in a chair with minimal support, or try to lay down to sleep!!

I try to avoid self-pity, but it was really hard to keep up the good face while I knew everyone else was much healthier and probably felt better. I grant that quite a few older folks there probably had arthritis or other chronic problems, but precious few have struggled with cancer for four years with no solution in sight.

Another really annoying thing that happened tonight was that I thought I could wear the gorgeous maroon silk-satin beaded blouse with the black moiré skirt. It's just stunning. I put it on and it fit — but my medi-port shows. Guess I'll never be able to wear it again. When the port is eventually removed, I'll have an unsightly scar.

I'm so sorry to complain to you like this, especially since there's really nothing you can do about it. This is my substitute for a phone call I guess, since you and Geordie are certainly asleep as I write. I hope your dinner party was a success — I'm absolutely sure it was. You'll have to share your menu with me as I don't remember asking about it yesterday.

I'm on my way back up to bed. I'll call you on Sunday.

Love you so much,
Mom

I read Mom's email with so many emotions: relief that she was still sharing her fears and frustrations with me; rueful, wishing that I hadn't been correct in assuming that her fears and frustrations were still there despite her strong front; incredulity that she still thought to ask about my dinner party when she felt so awful; and, finally, hesitant hope that we'd have good news to share with her soon.

That Saturday was the first time I could take an early indicator pregnancy test. I woke up early to take it, anxiously hoping to see the "+". I stood in the bathroom, staring at myself in the mirror as I waited to check the stick. After an interminable wait, I looked at the very clear "+" on the second line that indicated that I was pregnant.

"Geordie! Sweetie, wake up!"

"What time is it? Are you OK?" He mumbled as he half-sat up in bed.

"I'm sorry, it's really early, but I want to show you something. Close your eyes, I'm turning on the lights."

He covered his eyes as I flicked on the switch. I handed him his glasses and he blinked to get used to the brightness.

"Look at this. What do you see? A plus, you see a plus, don't you?"

"It looks like it, but it's a little faint. Does that mean what I think it does?"

"YES! Sweetie, we're going to have a baby!"

His face broke into a huge grin.

"Wow, it definitely seems like it. But, I don't want you to get your hopes up. Wait until the doctor does the test on Monday before you get too excited."

That weekend, I took four more pregnancy tests, each of which showed a plus sign, with varying intensity depending on the time of day. Our obstetrician confirmed it on Monday — we were going to have a baby!

We debated whether to call Mom with our exciting news. I really wanted to wait — only three weeks — to tell my family in person when we went to Virginia for Thanksgiving. Besides, the risk of miscarriage would decrease every week and I was still afraid of getting her hopes up in case I lost the baby.

Talking to her without divulging our news was agonizing. My pregnancy was the most exciting thing that had happened in my entire life, except for marrying Geordie, and I felt like I was betraying her by not telling her. It was even worse during conversations when she was particularly blue, which were more frequent these days.

One afternoon about a week after we found out, we had an especially tough conversation. Her CA-125 had gone up another 500 points to almost 4500. She sobbed on the phone that she was beginning to wonder about the point of continuing treatments and putting the family through all of the hassle and uncertainty just to live a couple more months — and those in pain.

"I started Taxotere this morning. I'm so tired of spending half of my time sitting in a chair watching poisonous chemicals leach into my body. Cyndi drove me, but I don't know why she takes the time; she must have something better to do besides sit and try to keep me amused. I tried to tell her not to come, although I really appreciate her being there with me, especially when the nurse told me my awful number. She was so nice; the nurses are always so nice, that it almost makes me sadder. I feel like I'm just sad all the time now."

I almost blurted out my news, hoping that it would give her a lift even though it couldn't make her pain go away, but knew that it wasn't the right conversation for such a revelation. Still, I couldn't wait until Thanksgiving; I didn't even want to wait another day.

When Geordie got home that evening, he agreed with my decision to tell my parents now. We sat down on the sofa together and called Dad at work. Without divulging the reason for our call, we asked him to conference Mom in. They were both surprised to hear from us together.

"Hi, guys. You're probably wondering why I asked Dad to conference us all in on a call together. Geordie and I have some news." I paused for a second, then exclaimed, "You're going to be grandparents; we're having a baby!"

I heard Mom gasp on the other end of the line, and knew she was starting to cry happy tears in Arlington just like I was in London.

"Oh, Karen, this is just incredible. This is the best news you possibly could have given us. Being a parent is the most precious gift in the entire world."

"It's such a miracle. I'm sorry I wasn't home in October, but I wanted to be here the entire month to try another round of Clomid — and it worked! We got pregnant the very first time I ovulated."

"It sounds to me like it was just meant to work this way. When is this precious bundle expected to be born?" Mom's voice was more energized than I'd heard it in weeks.

"Depending on which doctor's chart you believe, either the 12th or 14th of July. So we're having a Bastille Day baby! We've only known for a week and it's been agony not telling you, but we really wanted to wait and tell you in person over Thanksgiving. Needless to say, I have no will power."

The excitement in Mom's voice validated our decision to tell my parents early.

"Oh, I'm so happy to know now. Besides, we need to plan our Thanksgiving shopping activities. You'll need maternity clothes, and it's just possible that we could start looking for the best baby stores, so we're ready for later. Of course, I also need to dust off my sewing machine and see which of my old patterns I can find. I made such beautiful clothes for you kids; I can't wait to make them for my grandchild."

"It sounds like I should probably sign off and get back to work so you ladies can plan. Congratulations gal, and Geordie, this is really terrific."

"Bye, Cliff. I think you have the right idea. I'm going, too. Bye, Grandma and Grandpa."

With that, Geordie and Dad hung up and Mom and I stayed on the phone for ages talking about her grandchild in progress.

The excitement of our baby almost overwhelmed another project I'd been working on for months. One evening, the previous spring, I had gone to a Harvard alumni event at The Institute of Cancer Research, the UK's foremost cancer research organization. The ICR, as it was called, was located just one block from our flat in London. I learned that their scientists were the world leaders in cancer drug development, and had mapped more cancer genes than any other organization worldwide, among other notable achievements.

As it happened, the clinical oncologist who presented at the event was the leading ovarian cancer oncologist in the UK. He spoke on the ICR's work on ovarian cancer — including its development of Carboplatin, the drug that had been so effective for Mom prior to her allergic reaction.

A few days later, I met with Brenda Bachelor, an ICR fundraiser. At a nearby pub, we sat at wooden tables while I talked to Brenda about Mom's experience, and shared with her the conclusions from my Stanford research paper. Brenda was a handsome woman, just a decade younger than my mother. She immediately engaged me with her thoughtful manner, and helped me think of ways that I could support the ICR's scientists in their work.

Mom was happy for me when I told her about my meeting, but she was also worried that I was letting cancer become my life. I tried to explain to her that it was the first time, ever, that I felt like I could make a real difference in the world. If I could find the right inroad, working to eradicate ovarian cancer, or at least decrease its incidence and increase patients' survival rates, could become my *raison d'être*.

"I guess, but I just want you to do it because it interests you and not because you feel you need to for me. Don't you find the whole topic depressing and want to get away from it sometimes?"

I felt that way sometimes, but not like she did. I wasn't a patient; I could escape into the rest of my life. She only had her life by fighting cancer successfully every day.

With Brenda's help, I decided to host an evening to raise funds for research into "Silent Cancers", an umbrella term I'd created for those cancers, like ovarian, that have few obvious, early symptoms and are often diagnosed after the cancer has already spread. Beth Franklin, my new friend from the Junior League, generously offered to hold the event at her luxurious flat in Chelsea, overlooking the River Thames.

I sent invitations to more than a hundred former colleagues and old and new friends whom I hoped would come and support the ICR and not be put off by the invitation that "suggested" sending a donation in order to attend an event in a private home. I also included information about the symptoms of silent cancers, in hopes of raising awareness as well as funds.

With all of my excitement about our baby, final prepara-tions for the November 20th fundraising event happened in a blurred flurry of activity — baking canapés and desserts, buying wine and flowers. That evening, Geordie welcomed nearly fifty of our friends. He spoke of how proud he was of me for bringing everyone together and I was surprised when his voice broke a bit, just as it had at our wedding a year before. It was then that I realized that my work on this event really was important to him.

As Geordie introduced me, I stepped to the front of the room to speak. I'd been really nervous as I'd read over what I planned to say in the taxi on my drive over. But somehow, I was at ease when I finally stood in front of our friends and colleagues.

"I can't tell you what it means to have all of you here this evening. It's completely overwhelming.

"Many of you have asked if my mother would be here this evening. Unfortunately, she is in the U.S. undergoing chemotherapy. But she would be ecstatic to see all of you here. As most of you know, she and I have undertaken a project to write a memoir about our lives as ovarian cancer patient and daughter. I hope you will indulge me in reading a brief excerpt — less than five minutes, I promise! — from her writing about her initial diagnosis.

"It's a wonderful thing to be healthy. Although I had bouts of illness as a child, I've spent my entire adult life as a strong, healthy person. My husband, Cliff, and I have been extremely conscientious about taking lots of vitamins, maintaining a healthy diet and getting adequate sleep and regular checkups. So of course I didn't expect to ever get cancer …"

It felt natural, albeit a bit surreal, to be reading Mom's words to my friends. I'd read this section so many times, that I tried to read expressively, catching the eye of various friends in the audience, but without baring all the emotions I'd felt at the time. Then, I looked at Beth and saw tears in her eyes. Suddenly, my own emotions threatened to overcome me. I swallowed, took a deep breath, and finished reading the excerpt that Mom and I had selected for this evening.

"... *So, the diagnosis was cancer, but I wasn't sure I believed it. How could I get cancer when no one in my family had ever had it?! Besides, I was sure I was meant to live lots longer than my 54 years to date.*

"Fortunately for us, my mother has been with us for four years since that initial diagnosis. She had her first major surgery during Thanksgiving week 1999, so it seems fitting that we celebrate her 'anniversary' right before that same week four years later.

"Over these four years, my mother has had myriad treatments, including eight different series of chemotherapy. One of the chemotherapy agents which gave her the best results was Carboplatin, which was co-developed by The Institute of Cancer Research. As a result, I personally credit the ICR's oncology research for making it possible for us to be here celebrating this evening.

"In every donation that you, our friends, make to The Institute of Cancer Research in conjunction with this event, there are funds going directly to help more people celebrate for years after their initial cancer diagnoses."

Our friends' warm applause and support filled me with satisfaction, which stayed with me throughout the evening.

The next morning, the soles of my feet were bruised from an entire evening spent in high heels, but my spirits were soaring. I opened my email to see a congratulations message from a friend, which I forwarded to Mom. I read her response, especially the signature line, over and over that day as I readied our flat and our bags to go home for Thanksgiving week.

Subject: Re: An Evening of Fine Wines

Wow!! How very nice to be recognized by someone you obviously hold in high esteem. His remarks should not be taken lightly. You will never know who or how many folks may benefit in the future by your information shared last night, and to be passed on by the attendees to others they care for.

Dad and I are enormously proud of you as you know and grateful that you have chosen the "silent cancers" to direct your efforts. We'll chat more later in person — just one more day.

Love you so much,
Mom, the survivor

HOLIDAYS
November – December 2003

KAREN

My parents met us at the airport with huge hugs. Mom looked exhausted as usual these days, but happier than when I'd last seen her in September. The dark circles under her eyes seemed almost to accentuate their bright excitement. Dad and Geordie quickly retrieved our bags and we were soon on the road.

We drove straight from the airport to Mathews to see Drew and Lynda, and watch Lynda perform at Donk's. As always, Drew greeted me with a huge, feet-off-the-ground bear hug. The pressure on my pregnant chest almost knocked the wind out of me. I tried to mask my grimace with a smile.

"Hey, Rufer! Is Lynda ready for her show tonight?"

"Yeah, she's already over there, so you won't see her until after the show. We probably need to leave pretty soon too."

"Bummer. Well," I looked over at Mom, Dad and Geordie. There wasn't any way I could wait until after the show to share our news. They knew it too.

"I'd wanted to tell you and Lynda together, but I can't wait. You're going to be an uncle!"

Drew's face exploded in a giant, incredulous smile. He looked at me, then at Mom, Dad and Geordie and back at me.

"Are you serious? You're pregnant?"

"We certainly are!"

Geordie broke in, "Actually, Karen's pregnant, not me. Just in case you were wondering."

Drew laughed. "I don't know why women say that. I've never met a pregnant guy." He turned to Geordie and Dad. "Have you?"

They shook their heads as Mom and I smiled at each other. Drew glanced at his watch.

"I hate to say it, but, we should head over to Donk's. Does anyone want to ride over with me?"

"We will" I turned to my parents, " — if that's OK. Do you mind if we meet you there?"

"Absolutely not, have a good ride with Uncle Drew and we'll see you there."

In the cab of Drew's truck, Geordie and I shared the details of our baby's due date and our excitement about becoming parents. Then, he asked about Mom.

"I hate to change from such a great subject, but have you noticed that Mom's been a lot more tired lately? The last time she and Dad came down, she napped most of the morning on our sofa. I read the emails, but do you know any more about how she's doing than what Dad sends?"

"Not really. I mean, she isn't doing well — the cancer has definitely spread and she's taking some pretty atrocious medications, in addition to being back on chemo." I paused, not sure whether to say the next thing on my mind. "I gather from Dad that she really tries to rally when they come down to visit you guys. At home these days, she probably sleeps about 14–16 hours a day."

Drew was quiet, and his knuckles turned white on the truck's steering wheel. He took a deep breath before asking, "Have the doctors said anything about how long she might have left?"

My words caught in my throat as I answered him.

"I don't think they know. Her CA-125 has been stable for a couple of months, but I don't even know if it's possible for it to go higher than it already is. I guess the good thing is that her doctor's still giving her chemo. I would hope that she'd end the treatment if she didn't have some hope of it prolonging Mom's life."

The truck was quiet as we turned into the parking lot across from the theater.

"I won't talk about it anymore now that we're here, but I do want to say that it must help Mom so much to have a grandkid on the way. That's really great."

After the show, I drove with Drew and Lynda to dinner and shared our big news. We didn't talk more about Mom then, but I had a feeling that our earlier conversation weighed on Drew's mind through the evening.

Back at my parents' home on Monday, Mom went on the computer after breakfast to check her emails before we left for her blood test and shopping. She called out to me in the family room, "Your poor dad. I used to get so annoyed when he sent my medical updates for me, that now he sends them all to me for approval, even though I no longer care to see them before they go out."

So, her forward message was brief, as was Dad's update:

Subject: Oncologist Appointment

Happy Thanksgiving all!!
Vicki/Mom

...The doctor said that Vicki's shortness of breath,
nausea, and tiredness were probably due to a combination of the chemo and the antiviral medication...

The examination was good, with nothing to report. I was
assigned the responsibility of making sure that Vicki
drinks six to eight glasses of water every day. A classic
case of responsibility with no authority, but I'll try.

Love,
Dad/Cliff

An hour after we left the house, Mom's medi-port had
been pricked for her blood test and I was the most svelte
shopper at *A Pea In The Pod* Maternity.

"I don't even know where to start."

Mom smiled as she replied.

"Well, think about the clothes you usually wear, and
then consider that nearly everything you currently own
won't fit in a few months."

A very patient sales associate took armfuls of clothes
back to the dressing room for us as we shopped the entire
store before finally deciding that it was time to start trying
things on.

The dressing room was cavernous with a comfortable
chair for Mom. She smiled when I started to fasten the
"bump" pillow around my waist.

"I was about to say that this feels a lot like wedding gown shopping, except that you certainly weren't putting extra padding around your waist then."

"Does that mean that you might cry if you like what I try on?"

"Oh hush. You know, I just might. This is so fun."

It was fun. Some of the clothes were truly hideous, and some it was hard to imagine ever fitting unless it turned out that I was pregnant with triplets. But many of them looked reassuringly stylish. After a while, I had the clothes sorted into three categories: a select few items in the "definitely yes" group, an enormous stack of "maybes", and a substantial "definitely no" pile that we handed to the sales associate when she came to check on us.

Mom and I surveyed the two remaining selections.

"Wow, I'm at a complete loss. Do you mind if I try on some of the maybes again?" I asked.

"Go ahead, I'm perfectly comfortable here and you can buy me lunch after we're done."

"It's a deal. Do you really mean you'll let me buy you lunch?"

"No, I guess it was more a figure of speech. I meant we'll go to lunch after."

As we bantered back and forth, I tried some of the clothes again. I discarded several items and committed to a few others, but still ended up with an enormous pile of "maybes".

Mom rose from her chair and gathered the "yes" and "maybe" stacks in her arms.

"OK, why don't you get dressed while I give these to the sales associate?"

"Wait, I'm still deciding about those. Don't worry; I'll

be dressed in a sec and I'll bring them out when I've figured out what I'm buying."

"I'm sorry, but you must have misunderstood. I intend to utterly spoil your child, starting with its mother. We'll take both of these piles, with no ifs, ands, or buts."

I shook my head with a huge smile. This was a refreshing glimpse of Mom at her most indulgent.

"Thank you. I... we really appreciate it."

Mom smiled. "You are going to be a wonderful mother. I just couldn't possibly be happier for you. Being a mom has been the best job I've ever had."

I gave her a big hug.

"I just hope I can be the same kind of mother you are for us."

"Oh, you'll be much better. I'm sure of that. Have I told you that I decided what I want to be called?"

"No, I can't wait to hear." Mom had been talking about what her name would be for the new baby since we'd first told her the news.

"GG, for Grandma Greve. What do you think?" She was so excited.

"GG. I think that's a brilliant name. I can't believe you took so long to tell me!"

"Well, I just came up with it the other day. It isn't like we haven't had other things to talk about."

She was right. We filled that week talking, mostly about baby-related things, while Dad worked and Geordie watched ice hockey and football on TV.

Drew and Lynda drove up on Thursday and we all had Thanksgiving dinner at Aunt Cyndi and Eric's. Our celebration was helped by Mom's latest CA-125 test of 3762 — still a terrifyingly high number, but down 700 from early November. She positively glowed looking around at her family all together when we sat at the table. She raised her glass.

"I feel like I have so much to be thankful for this year. Would it be too predictable if I just said how…" We all helped her finish her sentence, as it was one we'd heard many times, "…wonderful it is to have everyone together."

"Well it is!" she exclaimed, realizing that she was being teased by everyone. "And next year we'll even have one more reason to be thankful."

Geordie and I flew back to London that weekend, and on Monday Mom resumed her chemotherapy and doctors' appointments. I got Thursday morning's update from Aunt Cyndi when I turned on my computer.

Subject: Vicki's Busy Day with the Doctors

Guys,

What a busy day! Vicki made a whirlwind tour of three doctors' offices today. Here's a report.

Chemo went uneventfully, which is a good thing. She mentioned that she is really tired and asked about the possibility of a transfusion. The nurse scheduled one for her and she had it today. This should really help her energy level. The bad news is that it looks like Vicki will lose some of her hair because of the chemo. She talked with Marilyn, a stylish fellow chemo patient, about a new source for wigs.

...Then we saw her internist about the swelling in her ankles. He called it "edema" and attributed it to past surgery and radiation. He said that there's been a lot of medical activity in the groin area and that obstructs the veins. Vicki should try to keep her feet up whenever possible and avoid staying in one position for too long a time — like in a car or airplane.

...The internist was very positive when Vicki mentioned her new eye doctor. Apparently, he knows and trusts him. Conveniently, they're both located on the same floor of the same building, so it was an easy commute to our next appointment.

Great news about Vicki's current vision! Her right eye is 20/20 and her left eye is 20/30! Woo hoo! But the news gets better. He says there is no active virus in her left eye at this time. Once the inflammation disappears, it's possible for her left eye to return to 20/20. No promises, but...

He was very, very surprised that the research center administered radiation without a biopsy... Interesting...

Let me know if you have any questions.
Cyndi

It was all good news, or what passed for good news these days. Then I saw an email Mom sent to the Second Saturday ladies with a "cc" to me:

Subject: Just call me GG

Ladies,

I can't contain myself any longer. Cliff and I are expecting our first grandchild on or about Bastille Day, July 14.

After nearly a year of fertility experts and medication, Karen got pregnant in October. She is now about ten weeks along and doing very well. An enormous shopping trip to *Pea in the Pod* at Thanksgiving also assured that she will look stylishly pregnant as soon as she begins to show. She's already wearing the new bras because, as you mothers know, the boobs go first. They are deliriously happy, as are we.

See you all at the tea next week.

Love you all,
Vicki

PS The GG is for Grandma Greve

I emailed her right back to tease her for telling the ladies so early. She replied immediately:

The target announcement date was for next Thursday afternoon at the Ritz Carlton. You're correct — I just couldn't wait.

Love you so much,
Mom (GG)

It made me so happy to open my computer to see emails signed "GG". Mom and Dad were due to come to London on the 20th, and I couldn't wait to see them.

I was out shopping on the Kings Road for Christmas stocking gifts when Mom called after her transfusion.

"Marilyn didn't make it."

Who? Then it occurred to me. She was Mom's fellow ovarian cancer patient who'd just recommended a new wig shop. Marilyn and Mom had shared countless chemo sessions over the past few years, and I remembered her as a vibrant woman about Mom's age.

"She seemed fine when I saw her just a week ago, and now she's gone. It could be like that for me too." Mom broke down and sobbed into the phone.

"Oh, Mom, I'm so sorry."

"I'm not ready to die yet. I thought I was, but I'm not. I have too much left to live for. I want to meet my grand-child and sew baby clothes. But I have so little energy; I sleep almost constantly. If you'd asked me who'd go first, between Marilyn and me, I'd have said me. She seemed in great shape. This is such an insidious disease."

I tried not to let Mom know that I was crying.

"Yes it is. But Mom, your doctor wouldn't be giving you chemo if she didn't believe it was helping you." Then I remembered that Mom had seen Marilyn at chemo just a week before. I don't know if she thought of it too; she didn't say anything.

"I guess. My entire life consists of needles and doctors right now. I hope it's all for some benefit because I'm so tired of this routine. I'm counting the days until I get to see you in London. Just four more days."

"Me too, Mom. I love you so much."

"I love you too. Take good care of that little baby for me. I'm still feeling pretty blue, so I think I'm going to sign off and just go have a good cry and a nap. It's that kind of day."

"Will you be OK? Do you want me to call Dad or Aunt Cyndi?"

"Cyndi was with me when I found out. I'll be fine; I just want to be alone for a little while. I'll talk to you soon."

I looked at all the shoppers around me, searching for the perfect gifts for people who, I was quite certain, wanted for nothing. The only gift I really wanted to find was anything that would cheer Mom, or miraculously make her healthy. Empty handed, I walked back home through Chelsea in a daze, stopping at Starbucks for my usual chai tea latte that today tasted too sweet for my melancholy. Back at home, I called Aunt Cyndi and Dad, just to be sure they were watching out for Mom given the precipitous dip in her spirits. Then, I curled up in the fetal position on our bed and cried until I ran out of tears. I lay there for a few more minutes before I started to feel disgusted by my self-absorbed melancholy. I got up and busied myself wrapping Christmas gifts until Geordie got home. The next day, I got Dad's next update email.

Subject: Vicki's Doctor Appointment

Vicki had an appointment with her oncologist this afternoon. She was very happy with the pelvic examination, saying that everything there looked fine. Vicki told her that she was in pain almost all the time and had no energy, even though she had had two transfusions in the last three weeks. The doctor said that first of all, we need to get control of the pain and prescribed a skin patch slow release pain medication ...

... She was surprised that the Topotecan was having such a devastating effect on Vicki. She suggested an MRI, which is scheduled for noon on the 29th, before the next round of chemo.

... Vicki asked what her prognosis was, in view of the other patient who recently passed away while seeming to be in great health. Her doctor said that the other patient was a different case than Vicki and that she was very sick but hid it well. She said that there was no way that she could predict anything about Vicki's case, since if the chemo holds the tumor in check, things could remain stable for a long time.

... We talked about the trip to London, and as long as the pain medication has started working, the doctor thinks there is no reason not to go.

Love,
Dad/Cliff

When our doorbell rang Saturday night, I buzzed my parents in, and then raced down the four flights of stairs to see them. Geordie followed behind me to help Dad bring in the bags. I engulfed Mom in a big hug and was shocked by how frail she felt in my arms. Geordie gave her a kiss on the cheek while I hugged Dad.

"I'm so glad you're both here. How was your flight?"

"We're so glad we're here too! And it was a very good idea for us to take the day flight. I'm really tired, but I feel much better than I would if we'd taken the red eye."

It was a relief to hear Mom talking about feeling better … than something. Geordie and Dad carried their bags into our flat. Once again, I was amazed by how many bags my parents had brought with them.

"Did Lynda and Drew send tons of things with you again? I'm so sorry that you guys have to work as Christmas camels bringing gifts back and forth."

"Actually, we just have a lot of gifts from everyone." Dad was in the kitchen getting drinks with Geordie, so Mom lowered her voice. "I'm afraid that a lot of the gifts are actually for me from your Dad. I really wish he wouldn't waste his money on gifts that I won't be able to use for very long."

There it was: her first allusion to her condition.

"Mom, Dad loves you very much and wants to give you nice things for you to enjoy — for as long as you can."

"It makes me happy just to be here with you."

We spent the first few days of our visit quietly at home, talking about the baby and looking at pictures of nursery furniture online. Mom napped several times each day, while Dad and I went for walks and runs around the neighborhood and in Hyde Park.

In addition to her fatigue, Mom had nearly stopped eating. We tried to arrange meals that she would eat, but nearly everything was too... something. The raisin walnut bread she usually loved to eat toasted with peanut butter was too hard to chew. Nearly every dinner was too spicy for her — even basil was too strong a flavor for her chemo-altered taste buds. We watched her struggle to force down some food each meal, and tempted her with ice cream every afternoon and evening.

On Christmas Eve, Mom, Dad and I went to the Royal Albert Hall for an afternoon Christmas Carol service, and then met Geordie at our little Anglican church for the early children's Christingle service. On Christmas morning, we sat around our brightly decorated tree that, true to Greve family tradition, had gifts spilling out far beyond the widest branches. That afternoon, I could tell that Mom was tired from a busy evening the night before and from opening all those gifts, but it seemed like a happy kind of tired.

Six months earlier, I had urgently left Bain afraid that Mom wouldn't be with us through the fall. I hadn't dared dream then that she'd still be here and able to travel to London this Christmas. I had the feeling that she was living her ninth life and desperately hoped that it would last long enough for her to meet her grandchild. Thinking about the baby seemed to keep her going. She smiled at me when I asked her questions about her own pregnancies, most of which started with, "How did you feel when ..."

"I'll try to remember for you, but there's something I need you to do for me. Whenever you think of a question you want to ask me, write down the question and your own answer to it. That way, in thirty years when your daughter is asking you how much weight you'd gained when you were twelve weeks pregnant with her, you'll know the answer."

"Touché. It's hard to believe I could ever forget all of these feelings, but I guess I will."

"You won't forget the most important ones, but memories do tend to evolve and get replaced over and over again as your kids grow up and do increasingly amazing things. You'll see; it's something I don't think you can understand until you're a mother yourself."

"I guess. It's hard to believe that I will be in July."

"Believe it; you'll be a mother before you know it. I can hardly wait."

She smiled in tired anticipation. Once again, I was grateful that she had a grandchild to look forward to.

DECLINE
January – February 2004

KAREN

My parents left on December 28th, and Geordie and I brought in the New Year in the true party spirit. We cuddled on the sofa to watch a movie and at a quarter to ten finally conceded that we were both exhausted. We'd been asleep for two hours when the clock struck midnight, and we woke up the next morning refreshed to start 2004.

My first order of business was to finalize my resignation from Bain. I'd appreciated the flexibility of my Leave of Absence during the fall, and now was ready to close that chapter in my life. My life was busy and fulfilling with my Junior League and ICR charity commitments, plus swimming and pregnancy yoga classes to keep fit for the baby.

My busy schedule helped me justify my long break from working on the book; the emotional reasons were harder to accept. I was struggling to come to grips with the reality that Mom was finished with her role of co-author. She hadn't written since one real-time bit late last summer about radiation; these days she struggled to write more than an occasional brief email. Our book was meant to be a shared endeavor. Without Mom, I couldn't care enough to write.

The other reason I wasn't writing was the same as the reason Mom wasn't writing. She was getting weaker every day. Once again, she had rallied all her energy around a big event — this time, Christmas in London. Each of Dad's emails and calls revealed that she was sleeping more, eating less, in greater pain, and having more side effects. I was too immersed in her present condition to write about what had happened before, and couldn't bring myself to write about her obvious decline.

I felt trapped between two devastating scenarios. The first was the uncertainty with which we'd lived for over four years, and which felt more torturous the closer my baby's due date came. The second was losing her. Every time I thought of this, my heart tightened and I couldn't breathe. I spent much of that January gasping for air, trying to get through the wretched premonition of losing Mom. The pregnancy yoga classes served a dual purpose for me: while others learned how to breathe during labor, I learned how to breathe every day that I came closer to losing my mother and best friend.

Dad started to email and call more and more to let us know how Mom was and what we could/shouldn't do. The engineer in him never would have considered journaling, but his emails kept us in the loop while recounting his losing battle to keep his wife happy and healthy.

Subject: Mom

I'm really concerned. I just can't get Mom to eat much at all. This morning she was 148 pounds, down from

165 before London. She says that the food doesn't taste good, but even when I get puddings, ice cream, and other things she likes, she might eat a couple of tablespoons before she says that she is full. She's had lots of anxiety attacks in the last couple of days, which Ativan seems to cure, and some breakthrough pain, which Dilaudid takes care of. The problem is that she is getting very weak, which is understandable given the weight loss and everything else that she is fighting. She's going to call her oncologist for an appointment today, to see if we can find out what is happening.

The last thing we want to do is lecture her on the necessity of eating, since it just makes her nervous. When I serve a meal, she just sits there for five minutes before she tries to start eating, and I know that she is psyching herself up, which makes it impossible to eat. I've had some luck sneaking Christmas cookies, Dove bars, puddings, et cetera in between meals, but she gets so nervous before the meal that she couldn't possibly eat.

... If you call her, don't talk long, because she doesn't have much strength, and holding the phone takes energy. She would probably like to hear from you, just for encouragement.

Love you all,
Dad/Cliff

Subject: Snow

We got about one inch of VERY slippery snow last night. Things are really bottled up today, but I'm sure that everything will be gone before Drew and Lynda come up tomorrow.

… Mom is at the hospital getting a transfusion. I took her over, and Cyndi is going to pick her up. She was really run down last night, and didn't eat much this morning, but she said that she gained a little weight back, so things are going in the right direction. Love you all.

Dad/Cliff

I couldn't focus after getting this email, so I called Dad at the office.

"Hi Dad, I just got your email. How are you doing?"

"Oh, I'm fine. The snow is really just more of a nuisance than anything."

"That's good. Actually, I was more wondering how you were doing with everything with Mom? I'm really worried about how much worse she seems than when you were here for Christmas."

"Well, that trip took a lot out of her, but hopefully this transfusion will give her more energy. I just wish I could get her to eat."

I took a deep breath, not wanting to say what was really on my mind.

"Dad, we asked my doctor and she confirmed that I'm not supposed to fly transatlantic after I'm 28 weeks pregnant, and then until the baby is at least a month old. That means no flights to DC between about mid-April and mid-August."

"I think you'd mentioned that before, and it makes sense. I'm really glad you're coming in February and April. I'm afraid I don't think Mom can fly there anymore, but she's looking forward to your visits."

"Me too."

I wiped angrily at the tears that wouldn't stay away.

"Actually, the reason I mentioned this spring is that if Mom takes a bad turn, or we lose her, I won't be able to fly home."

I paused to blow my nose. I couldn't believe we'd gotten to the point where we were discussing my final visit to see Mom.

"I've thought a lot about it and talked to Geordie. One possibility is for me to come there for my third trimester and have the baby in DC. The thing is, I just can't stand the thought of being away from him for those three months or risk him not being there for our baby's birth."

"No, that makes sense. You should be there with Geordie and your doctors in London."

"The other possibility I've looked into, if anything should happen after my no-fly date, is taking a ship back. The Queen Mary cruise ship only takes six days from Southampton to New York. It's quite expensive, since most people use it for holiday rather than for transportation, but it's an option that could make sense."

It was Dad's turn to pause as he considered my information.

"That's an option that hadn't occurred to me. Let's hope it doesn't come to that. But, you should know that Drew and I have talked about the possibility that Mom might pass away when you can't travel. We both feel that we would wait to have her memorial service until you could come home for it with the baby. Vicki wants to be cremated anyway, so there's no rush to have the service right away. We don't want this to be something that worries you."

Tears were flooding down my face now.

"Dad, I can't tell you what that means to me. Hopefully we won't have to deal with any of it, but I really appreciate you and Drew thinking about this for me. I feel so lucky that we have such a strong family through this whole ordeal. I'm amazed by how well we're all sticking together."

"We don't exactly have a choice, but you're right. I guess that's really something that Vicki has helped to teach us all. I'm sorry to cut you off, but I have to get to a meeting. Have a good day gal; I love you."

"I love you too, Dad. Thanks again for being so understanding. Have a good rest of the day."

A week later, Mom missed her Second Saturday breakfast with the ladies. It was the first time in over four years that she was in town, but just didn't have the energy to go.

I still called her at least once each day, striving to end our conversations before she seemed too tired — and to talk about happy things. Our phone conversations resembled an emotional lottery. Sometimes, she sounded great, full of energy and enthusiasm for her activities and the baby. Later the same day, she might sound dejected and exhausted, and end the call after a few minutes.

During our best conversations, we talked about the baby, including our nursery that Mom insisted on furnishing for us. I sent her an email with six links to various websites that pictured strollers, cribs, basinets, and other nursery furniture. Her response was the first email I'd gotten from her in nearly a week.

Subject: Re: nursery!

Imagine my surprise to find a web site that actually shows pictures of furniture. These were more to my liking. Hope that we can actually find some things here. I'd forgotten just how much fun this can be.

I opened her email first thing in the morning and waited until early afternoon to call her. We had the best conversation we'd had in ages, talking about various nursery options. She sounded great and I desperately hoped that she was on the upswing.

Subject: Re: Vicki's appointments 1/20/04

I'd like a copy of what Dad sent to everybody on Tuesday. Somehow, I didn't get the original message.

This was the first time Mom had taken an interest in her medical update emails in a long while. I took it as another sign that she was feeling better. I was eagerly anticipating my upcoming visits: two in February and another in April for Dad's 60th birthday, just before my 28 week cut-off from flying.

I didn't talk to her much the next week; she didn't seem to have much energy and I was swamped with Junior League work before my trip. So I was caught off-guard by Dad's email.

Subject: Mom

As you have probably noticed if you talked to Mom over the last couple of days, she has become pretty incoherent. I don't know what is happening. Her medication is the same, in fact, I have been getting her up at five in the morning to take her first pill so that they are evenly spaced …

Since she has chemo tomorrow, I called the chemo nurses and asked them to observe her. The oncologist may want Vicki to have a head MRI to check for brain tumors, which are a possibility with ovarian cancer metastasis. Just wanted you all to know that we are trying to find out what is happening, without alarming Vicki. She doesn't know that I called her doctor.

Dad/Cliff

Two days later, things were looking up a bit.

Subject: RE: Mom

Hi! Things have improved. We reduced one of her medications and Vicki was much, much better last night. She slept all day yesterday, literally, which may have had something to do with it, but she was coherent and alert. This morning she was really mad at me for calling the doctor yesterday, which indicates that she's back to normal. She wouldn't have cared the way she was before.

I hope that the problem was just overdosing on the narcotics. This is strong stuff, so overdoses can really put her under. Let's hope.

Dad/Cliff

The next day, I anxiously scanned the crowd for my parents when I exited the U.S. Customs doors. There was Dad in a flannel shirt, standing near a set of chairs and waving for me. Where was Mom? I started to choke back tears with the realization that she hadn't come. Then Dad turned around and I finally noticed Mom sitting in one of the chairs near him. He helped her stand as I walked over to them and collected my hugs and kisses.

Mom looked much weaker even than she had just five weeks earlier in London. She probably shouldn't have come with Dad to pick me up. But my relief that she was still well enough to go to the airport to meet her daughter stayed with me throughout the drive home.

We all went to bed early that night; I was tired from my flight and my parents, especially Mom, were just tired. Dad came in to hug me good night, and to remind me to take it easy with Mom.

"I know you guys have a lot planned, and she's really looking forward to it. But you have to take it really easy. She has to nap each day, and she can't walk very much."

I couldn't blame him for the reminder, and was really worried about how to do even part of what we'd planned. But, being us, we managed to fit in the most important things, namely loads of medical appointments counterbalanced with a bit shopping.

Mom insisted on starting with a shopping trip on Sunday to buy my birthday present — an obscenely expensive new purse. I saw a glimpse of her old enthusiasm as she fingered the black leather and said, "I never thought I would be able to afford to buy a Louis Vuitton bag. I love buying you nice things."

"You've bought most of my nicest things. Mom, thank you for this purse. It's just gorgeous, and so decadent that I know I shouldn't have it, but I love it."

"Then it shall be yours." Her eyes grew misty and her chin wrinkled as she added, "Who will buy you nice things when I'm gone?"

I put my hand on hers as we each bit our lips to try to stop our tears. We had so many of these moments now, and it was reassuring to share these emotional fissures. I was certain that we each still had more crying sessions alone than together. With my new purse in one hand and her hand on my other arm, we walked slowly back to the car to go home and rest.

On Monday morning, Mom had her brain MRI. After an afternoon nap, she decided that a good reward would be to go look at nursery furniture. This excursion served as my critical reminder that we couldn't walk too much. We parked as close as we could to the baby superstore, but she was still tired just from crossing the outlet mall parking lot. We decided to check out the glider chairs first and sat next to each other as we surveyed the floor, discussing our ideal crib, glider chair, changing table, linens, lamps and other essentials for the perfect nursery. Since none of it could be shipped to London, her only purchase comprised two multi-colored plastic balls with perfect grips for a baby's little hands. She bought one for our baby and one for Anne-Marie's, due in August.

On Tuesday, Mom saw Carter at noon, followed by her eye doctor. Then, we came home and each took afternoon naps before going to her oncologist's office for Procrit. The chemo nurses were as friendly and concerned as ever, greeting my mom and me with warm, comforting hugs.

I remembered my initial discomfort with what I'd perceived as the nurses' overly affectionate manner with patients. Now, two years later, it suddenly made sense. Watching Mom as she sat in the chair, mouth wide open to breathe more easily, eyelids too heavy to open more than half-mast, I realized that she was a pale shadow of the newly-retired CPA who'd first come to this clinic. The only thing that hadn't changed during her decline was how the nurses treated her. When she had walked in briskly, bursting with wedding or holiday pictures and stories to share, they had greeted her with warm hugs and caring smiles. Now, when she slowly shuffled across the room in her slippers to collapse exhausted into a chair, she received the same warm hugs and caring smiles. I was especially grateful to Mom's nurses when I had this epiphany.

On Thursday, our only commitment was to go shopping for my bump. I needed clothes for a couple of upcoming events, and Mom sat with me in the same maternity dressing room where she'd indulged me so extravagantly at Thanksgiving. This time was more realistic than our visit at seven weeks, as I now knew that my belly wasn't the only part of me growing with the baby. After buying two dresses, we left the store. Conveniently situated across the mall corridor was a baby clothes boutique.

Mom looked at me with a grin, and I smiled back at her. "Shall we take a little look?"

We walked through the store, fingering little girls' smocked dresses and little boys' shirts and shorts. "I know you didn't want me to buy anything when we were here during Thanksgiving, but do you think GG could buy a little something for her grandchild now?"

"What would GG have in mind? It's hard, isn't it, not knowing if it's a boy or a girl. We have our scan scheduled just before my next visit, if you want to wait until then."

"How about if I buy one outfit now that could be for a little girl or boy, and then more clothes later when we know?"

We selected a darling little white long-sleeved "onesie" with blue and red stars on the collar, a matching red brimmed hat with a white ribbon, and white socks with blue and red stars. It felt right that Mom bought our baby's first outfit.

Friday, we had lunch with Aunt Cyndi, and then went to the clinic for Mom's chemo. On Saturday morning, I flew back to London. It was my first time taking the day flight instead of the red eye, and I spent much of the flight thinking about the past week. It had felt so long and yet not nearly long enough.

Each morning, Mom needed several wake up calls to rouse herself for breakfast with Dad, which she still refused to miss, though she hardly ate anything. She fell asleep as soon as he left each morning, waking up in time for her first appointment of the day only with prodding from Aunt Cyndi or me. Sometimes, she was her witty, vibrant self, but increasingly she seemed disoriented and confused. She was always tired, always in pain, and usually sad. She cried so much on Friday, it was heartbreaking.

For the first time, I felt like this visit was as much for Dad as for Mom, and I didn't get nearly as much time alone with him as I would have liked. I felt like I was abandoning him when I left for London, even as I looked forward to the break to reinvigorate myself before my next visit. I was acutely aware that he never got a break; I was developing a new level of admiration for Dad as he lovingly cared for Mom while watching her decline.

On February 18th, Geordie met me at the hospital for our twenty week ultrasound scan. I clutched his hand nervously as the technician moved the wand over my bulging belly. She noted that the baby's heart and brain were developing well, and commented that the baby was tucked right down in my pelvis.

"Can you tell if it's a boy or girl?"

"I could make a guess, but the baby really isn't in a position where I can see clearly. I can tell you that I think I see little boy bits, but it isn't clear enough to be sure. I'll need you to come back anyway to finish looking at the baby's spine, so hopefully I can tell you then."

Geordie set our appointment for two weeks later while I tried to control my tears. I'd so desperately hoped to be able to share our baby's gender with Mom during my upcoming visit, to give her a little lift. From Dad's updates, it seemed that she had declined even in the two weeks since my last visit.

Subject: Vicki's Doctor Appointment

We asked the oncologist about the dizziness, occasional disorientation, shortness of breath, and numbness in her arms and feet. These are caused in part by a combination of the narcotics interacting with the antidepressants, but are primarily because of her low blood oxygen level. The transfusion may help, but when she gets tired she just needs to rest. Her body is using most of its resources to fight the cancer. She should not drive because of the narcotics she is taking.

…In the exam, the doctor said that she was very encouraged by evidence of response. She had said earlier that stability and maybe a little response was all that we could hope for, so this was very encouraging. The CA-125 was not back, but she expected that it would be a little lower based on the exam. Gaining weight and eating more are signs that the Topotecan is having some effect.

Her next appointment is in four weeks. She'll get two pints of blood tomorrow, and chemo again next week. Cyndi and Vicki will get the new handicapped sticker for the car today. All in all a very good check up.

Love,
Dad

So, this was what now passed for "a good check up". When I arrived at the airport on Sunday, I wasn't surprised to see Dad alone. It had finally happened, the first time Mom's cancer had kept her from meeting me. I gave him a big hug and tried to talk to him on the drive home about what was happening with him, before catching up about Mom. That part of our conversation was brief. Work was going well, and his colleagues were being incredibly understanding about his need to stay in DC rather than travelling to customers and subcontractors as he usually did almost weekly.

His update on Mom wasn't as upbeat as his email had been. After stabilizing around 3500-3700 from November to January, Mom's February CA-125 was up nine hundred points, to 4680. I wondered aloud how high it could go, and he shook his head. He admonished me to be sure she rested as much as possible, and to try to give her food whenever she would accept it. His latest trick was to make milkshakes with ice cream. Apparently, Mom really liked them and had several small shakes daily, with a straw to make drinking easier. She also loved mini Dove ice cream bars and ate several each day.

Mom was asleep on the family room sofa when we came in, wearing her nightgown and bathrobe and covered with an afghan.

"Hi."

She stirred when she heard us and smiled weakly, putting her hand out to take mine. "I'm sorry I didn't come to get you. How was your trip?"

"Hi, Mom," I gave her a kiss on the cheek. "My flight was fine, and I'm glad you didn't come to the airport — you needed to be here resting. We have plenty of time this week to spend together. Now let's all get up to bed."

"Okay, twist my arm." She replied with a smile, and put out her arm for me to help her to sit up, and then turned to rise from the sofa. She leaned heavily on me to stand, and shuffled slowly to the stairs, and then up to her room, stopping a few times on the way. She seemed a decade older than she had on my last visit, just two weeks before.

On Monday, Mom napped intermittently throughout the day, and then kept me company while I made lasagne — one of her old favorites — for dinner.

The next day, I drove her to Carter's, then brought her back home and made lunch. She picked hesitantly at her food, and then said, "This is wonderful, but I'm not really hungry right now. Do you mind terribly if I just lie down on the sofa here for a little nap?"

"Not at all. Do you want anything from the mall? I have a lot of little errands I should run and I'm happy to pick a few things up for you if you'd like."

"The only things I really need are new bras. Mine just don't fit anymore. But is that something you can really buy me?"

"Why don't I buy a selection and bring them back for you to try on."

I tucked her in and gave her a kiss. "I'll be back in a little while."

It felt odd to walk around the mall without Mom, as trips here had been a mainstay of my visits home for years now. She was my favorite shopping companion and I had to bite my lip walking by the baby store where she'd bought our baby's little outfit, realizing that she might not be back there again.

Mom looked at the bras when I got home, but didn't want to try them on.

"I'm sure they're fine. I'll try them when I need to wear them."

She sat up on the sofa and I made her a milkshake.

"Will you help me with a project I'm planning? Drew and I are going to make Dad a special album for his 60th birthday that chronicles his life so far."

I saw Mom get a gust of energy. "What a lovely idea. That's just the sort of thing I'd like to help with. Go get the albums from the credenza in my office and we'll look through them together."

We spent the next hour savoring family albums, as I promised repeatedly to scan the pictures I wanted to use and keep the albums intact. Mom traced the pictures with her finger, recalling the memories of her and Dad's wedding, and Drew's and my early years.

"You were such wonderful kids. Your father and I couldn't be luckier."

"We're pretty lucky ourselves. I love you so much."

"Me too. More than you could ever know. Do you mind if we switch gears for a while and look at more pictures later? I want to show you the recipe for chicken salad I'd like you to make for the Commonwealth Circle luncheon on Thursday."

"Of course, which cookbook is it in?"

"I knew you'd ask that."

"Well, it will be hard to make it without the recipe, don't you think?"

"Smart aleck. I think it's in ..." On about the tenth attempt, we found the recipe in one of her hundred plus cookbooks. I made the casserole on Wednesday as she oscillated between sleeping and giving me instructions from the sofa.

Mom had wonderful friends and I was looking forward to seeing them at the luncheon on Thursday, even though I wasn't sure until we actually left that we'd really be going. It was the first time all week that Mom had squeezed her feet into real shoes, in lieu of the comfortable moccasin-style slippers she'd been wearing indoors and out. She even put on makeup for the occasion and looked the best I'd seen her in months.

Mom rallied as only she could and spent two hours socializing and laughing with her friends. In addition to five of the six Second Saturday ladies, there were about twenty other women, many of whom were also past members of the Junior League of Northern Virginia. Nancy, Willie, Jean, and Claire from the Second Saturday group each separately approached me to say how wonderful Mom seemed — the best they'd seen her in weeks. She was in rare form — swapping stories energetically and even eating most of a plate of food. It was a refreshing glimpse of the "old" her.

On Friday, Mom had chemo, and then Drew and Lynda drove up after work to visit for the night. Drew and I stayed up until four o'clock in the morning poring through family photo albums and thousands of loose prints for Dad's birthday album. While I scanned the pictures into the computer and saved them to disk, we talked and laughed about our shared memories. Drew and Lynda's visit helped Mom to maintain Friday's enthusiasm until she and Dad dropped me at the airport Saturday evening.

It was a relief to be back in London with Geordie. I hated being away from him at any point, but the worse Mom's health was, the harder it was to go days without being able to talk to him in detail, which the time change and his job made impossible. We went for a long walk on Sunday after I shared details of my week in Virginia. This was so hard.

COMMUNICATIONS
Early March 2004

KAREN

Our family email traffic from early March exemplified our constant focus on Mom and her treatment. Those from Dad and Aunt Cyndi made me grateful for what they were doing for her, guilty for not being there to help, and almost more guilty for feeling grateful for my reprieve. I worried that it didn't make sense for me to wait until Dad's birthday in April to go back to DC. Each email I read or conversation I had seemed to validate this concern.

> Subject: Mom
>
> I'm afraid that I made Mom really mad at me today, in addition to adding to her frustrations. I asked if she had had a chance to call KPMG to get them to send her a W-2 so we can file our taxes ... She got mad and suggested that I call KPMG myself.

There are a ton of things falling in cracks, but the only things I'm pushing on are things that are really important, like sending the check for her life insurance so that it doesn't lapse (one of the three bills we have had over a week unpaid). She is getting really huffy around me, and nothing I do is right. I understand her frustration, but it's tough to take. Sorry for venting ...

Dad/Cliff

_____

Subject: RE: Mom

Dad, I'm so sorry about Mom's reaction to your conversation. I don't know if it's possible to get the balance right between taking care of things and not letting her feel like she's being handled or controlled. For the record, I think you're doing it as well as you possibly could.

Aunt Cyndi, thanks for taking her to her appointment tomorrow ...

That's all for now, except that I love you both very much and am so appreciative of how well you are taking care of Mom. She's lucky to have such a great family team.

Love, Karen

_____

Subject: RE: Mom

Guys,

For the record, Vicki was upset, but I think she's fine now. I think the hardest thing for her right now is trying to reconcile wanting to maintain control over normal daily activities with her inability to complete those activities. For example, her mind wants to be in charge of contacting KPMG for that W-2. Unfortunately, her body simply wouldn't allow it today.

When I arrived at the house today at noon, Vicki was fast asleep on the sofa, still in her nightgown and bath-robe, with the phone on her stomach … It took her a while to wake up and I had to physically help her sit up when she was ready. All day, she maintained a sort of eyes-at-half-mast look and had a hard time keeping on topic in conversations. Cliff, is it possible that she took a second pill by mistake? It seemed a lot like the time that she was overmedicated …

We had a quiet afternoon together while I ironed fabric for a new quilt. She's already told me that she really enjoys playing with fabric, even if I'm the one actually doing the work. The fabric really lifts her spirits. Around four, I made Vicki a milkshake (she drank a whole glass!) and made sure she was OK for me to leave.

… I don't think she should have anything on a list for her to do unless it's a fun activity. Cliff, this is not a dig at you. I know that she wants to maintain control and that you are in a no-win situation. The trick will be convincing her to spend her time doing fun things instead of paying bills and making phone calls …

Also, I'm not sure she's in any condition to go to her appointment tomorrow. Today was the worst I've seen her … she didn't venture beyond the kitchen and foyer … I'll try to make the call tomorrow when I see her. Maybe she can take Carter's appointment on the phone …

Thanks, guys, for the support. I'm sorry this is so long, but I'd rather err on the side of too much information.

Love you all,
(Aunt) Cyndi

Subject: RE: Mom

Hi guys,

Aunt Cyndi's experience yesterday sounds like most of the days I was there last week. I had the distinct impression each day that if I hadn't been sitting next to her on the sofa talking to her and helping her up, sometimes with this process taking 30 minutes, she would have stayed there asleep until Dad came home for dinner. To be honest, this even happened on days when she wasn't taking any supplemental medicine. I found it to be more related to the stimulus she was receiving.

During "highs" like the Commonwealth Circle luncheon and Drew and Lynda's visit, she rallied considerably and was much more engaged and lucid than other times.

Speaking of this, she has a Garden Club tea tomorrow afternoon for which she was to take tea sandwiches. I don't know whether she wants to go, but if she does, she'll need sandwich help. If not, you may need to help her remember to decline ...

Thanks to both of you. I'm sorry I'm not still there to help. Please write to update or vent anytime — it really helps me to stay involved and informed.

Love, Karen

———————————

Subject: RE: Mom

I took over the checks last night, so they are all paid. Vicki told me that there were only two. When I went through the stack of mail, I found (unopened) a mortgage bill, the car insurance bill, a utility bill, a cable bill, and several others. All of these were very close to the due date. I didn't go into details with Vicki except that there were other bills she hadn't opened. Vicki told me, when I started to pay the bills, that if I paid the bills she would not write any more checks. I said that was fine. I guess the case is closed.

Vicki told me this morning that she feels out of control,

that everyone is controlling her life. I told her that we were just trying to help her do things so that she could conserve her strength. She said that she understands that she doesn't have the energy to do things, but that she hates to live that way. This is just a tough time, and it's not going to get better …

I think her grogginess is mostly due to lack of oxygen. Her heart, without stimulation, probably doesn't pump enough blood to keep her brain alert. I'm due to give her Procrit tonight, which may give her a boost.

Well, enough of my ramblings, and I have to do some work for this company. Love you all, and thank you so much for all the help.

Dad/Cliff

———————————

Subject: Today's Update (March 2, 2004)

Guys,

Starting today, I'm planning to be with Vicki pretty much every day. I have been, but this makes it official. Given that, I'm also going to send out an update each evening. I'll try to keep them brief, but I thought this might keep everyone connected and up-to-date.

Vicki was upstairs in bed when I arrived this morning at 10:45. She required more time and help getting ready this morning and we didn't leave for Carter's office until 11:55 am (her appointment was at noon). We were very late, but Carter gave her a generous amount of time. Carter also gave me her home number and told me to keep her updated. What a giving person! I suggested that when Vicki is this tired that we could have her appointment by phone. Carter said that she could come to Vicki's house. Wow. I think we should look into that ...

Once we were home, Vicki stayed awake for about twenty minutes before it was nap time. She slept really hard (through the phone ringing numerous times) and didn't know it when I left around six this evening.

Tomorrow, we're scheduled for a tea with one of her clubs. We're taking tea sandwiches (more egg salad, anyone?) and shouldn't stay too long ...

All for now. Talk with you tomorrow.

(Aunt) Cyndi

_____

Subject: RE: Mom

Karen,

I love you. Don't worry about the bills; I was just venting a little. Mom was feeling pretty chipper this morning, and was even joking a little. Last night she was really bad; could hardly get her upstairs for bed. It just comes and goes.

I hope that everything is going well … Got to work now. Love you.

Dad

_____

Subject: Thank You

Cyndi,

… Thanks so much for all of your support. I really appreciate your planning to spend each day with Vicki, but please let me know if you can't do it, or have something else that you would like to do, because I can certainly work from home or take some time off to make sure that someone is with Vicki most of the time.

Are you going to chemo with her on Friday, or should I? If you go to chemo, you might want to talk with the nurses relative to whether we should be getting hospice involved at any point soon. I'm concerned that, once she can no longer do the stairs (which last night I was afraid would be this morning) we will need more help that one person can provide.

Cliff

_____

Subject: Re: Thank You

Cliff,

Actually, can you take Vicki to chemo on Friday? We're
headed to the Outer Banks and it would be great to
leave as close to noon as possible. That would also
give you the chance to talk to someone there about
oxygen, extra Procrit, and hospice …

As far as hospice goes, that's a really hard call. Forgive
my bluntness, but has Vicki's oncologist talked to you
in terms of time frames? Hospice isn't called in until the
end and I haven't heard that we're there yet. I understand that we might be, but I'm wondering if you've
heard something that I haven't. I'm also concerned that
Vicki knows what hospice is and that might squash
some of her hope, however unfounded it might be …

Cyndi

_____

Subject: Update for Wednesday, March 3

Guys,

Today was a good day.

… I arrived at her house this morning at 10:45 and Vicki
was showered and dressed! She had most of a bowl
of tomato soup and half a piece of toast for an early

lunch. Then we made sandwiches from egg salad and blanched asparagus spears for today's tea party. Vicki was tired but engaged in the process. She supervised closely and I assembled. We found a very nice glass platter and put the leftover spears in a small Delft vase in the center. Geordie, these details are for you. :)

She was tired by the time of the tea, but it was clear that she wanted to go. We arrived early and she took her place as one of the hostesses standing in the receiving line, though she was tired part way through and had to sit down. By the end of the meeting, she had fulfilled her responsibilities and spoken with some of her friends.

She received a beautiful floral arrangement this afternoon from Carole, which first made her cry and then perked her up. I left about 4:45 when Cliff got home.

That's all for now. Love you all,
(Aunt) Cyndi

Subject: Today's Update: Thursday, March 4th

By the way, today's the only date during the year that's also a sentence. :)

Guys,

… I want to share an episode that happened this

afternoon. The phone rang and we missed the call. The machine in the office took a message, which I could hear was a solicitor. Anyway, Vicki spent a full twenty minutes on the phone. I'm not sure how, but somehow she wound up talking to a telephone operator, learning about *69, and repeating, "I just want to know who called." Frankly, it was sad to watch. I'm guessing it was the medication talking.

After the phone thing, we went up to the sewing room, where Vicki slept for about three and a half hours. I left around five thirty.

For anyone who needs to know, Cliff will take Vicki to her chemo tomorrow morning. Then, around four thirty tomorrow afternoon, Nancy and Carole will bring Vicki tea.

By the way, I was talking with Karen this morning about a book that I'm reading. It's written by two hospice nurses and addresses quite directly how to best help patients … In some cases, I feel good knowing that I'm doing the right thing. In others, I need to reevaluate how I handle some conversations. Cliff, it deals directly with anger and might help you to understand better why she lashes out at you and how you might be able to defuse the situation … The writing style is easy to read even if the subject matter is not.

Take care. I'll email again on Monday.

(Aunt) Cyndi

In addition to our frequent emails, I spoke to my parents and Aunt Cyndi each day. My conversation with Mom that Saturday clinched my decision to go home early and prompted me to work on our book for the first time in months:

March 6, 2004

Earlier this afternoon, I called Mom and got a bad connection when she answered. I tried again and it was bad again so she said she'd call me. I waited 10 minutes before trying her back. The answering machine on the second line picked up, so I figured she was on the phone. The same thing happened five minutes later. On my third, attempt, she answered. She made no mention of not calling me back. Clearly, she'd forgotten to hang up the phone and also forgotten that she was going to call.

"So Mom, what have you been doing today?"

"I bought some new bras. My old ones didn't fit — the ones I got in London, so I needed some new ones."

I was surprised, since I'd just bought her new bras during my last visit.

"Oh, are these better than the ones I got you when I was home?"

"Yes, I think they're better for me. They fit pretty well."

"Oh, well that's good. Did Dad take you shopping to buy them?"

"No, that's not really his type of thing. I went by myself."

She's right that it isn't Dad's type of thing. But she can't drive anymore — she hasn't driven for over a month. Odd. I decide to move on.

"What's Dad been up to, then?"

"He's hard at work on something in the basement. He already went to the grocery store this morning. You know him, getting stuff done."

"I sure do. What do you have going on this afternoon?"

"Well, I need to go shopping for groceries. Unless Dad went, which I don't think he did. He might have." She paused. "But it doesn't look like it."

I try to digest the fact that she had just directly contradicted what she'd said less than a minute earlier. Then, I tell her a bit about my last few days.

"I found a good source of maternity bras here that are actually moderately priced! I just bought a few."

"Oh, and you bought me my new bras that I'm wearing now. I still need to pay you for these."

"Don't worry about it. I left the receipt on the counter with a deposit I asked Dad to make. Are you still wearing them with your other new ones?"

"These are my new ones. They fit fine."

It's her second direct contradiction of the conversation. I should be used to it by now — having her contradict herself, ask the same question five times in as many minutes, or misremember events or details. But it's the first time that she's fabricated activities she's done or will do. Does she wish that she could still shop by herself, even for mundane items like bras or groceries? Or is her mind just trying to fill the holes of the questions I'm asking? Where are the new bras from? I can't remember, but I must have bought them. What are you doing today? Well, Cliff's home, so it must be the weekend. I often go grocery shopping on weekends.

Whatever the reason, it's still hard to take. Geordie patiently turned down the volume on the football match on TV and listened as I recounted the conversation. I sat restlessly next to him for a couple of minutes before realizing that I had to get this one conversation, at least, if not the myriad others like it, down for the book so I'd remember it as it happened.

Earlier today, I tried to explain to him how overwhelmed I felt. I listed my commitments with the Junior League, The Institute of Cancer Research, Dad's birthday album, getting ready for the baby, and our personal finances. Writing about our conversation, I realize that I hadn't mentioned the biggest stress of all: the uncertainty surrounding Mom.

When Dad called the next Monday morning, I assumed it was in response to my email about coming home earlier for my next visit. It wasn't.

He was calling at the crack of dawn from the hospital, where he'd checked Mom in the night before. Her legs, particularly her right one, had swelled so badly that she wasn't able to stand up at all, much less walk. She could hardly breathe and was the least coherent she'd been so far. It turned out that she probably had a blood clot in her leg, and would be in the hospital for at least a few days.

"Before I even knew you'd taken her to the hospital yesterday, I sent you an email this morning that I want to come home this weekend. Now, I think I should move it up to Wednesday. I'll just schedule a trip through your birthday. I could come home even earlier, but Geordie and I have an ultrasound scan scheduled for tomorrow morning that I really want to do. For one thing, if our little one cooperates, we'll find out the sex and be able to tell Mom."

"I think it's a good idea for you to come home early, but don't worry about coming before your scan."

"Are you sure? You'd tell me if you thought," I paused,

"if I needed to be there earlier, wouldn't you?"

"I would, but she seems better this morning with whatever medication they're giving her. She's lucid enough that she asked me about plans for my birthday, which is a good sign."

"That is a good sign. Let me know how she's doing later today and I'll call tomorrow after our scan."

"Sounds good, gal. I love you."

"I love you too, Dad. Thanks for taking such good care of Mom."

I called Geordie to tell him about Mom's condition and that I would definitely be going back to DC on Wednesday, then spent most of Monday cramming in all of the calls, emails, bills, Junior League work and errands that I'd thought I had the next three weeks to deal with.

On Tuesday morning, our scan confirmed what our two previous ultrasounds had hinted at. We were having a baby boy! I could hardly wait to get out of the hospital in London to call Mom at the hospital in Virginia.

"Hi Dad. Is Mom awake and coherent enough to talk? If she is, is there a way that we can talk to you both at once?"

Dad replied in a cheerful voice that indicated that Mom was both awake and waiting for our call.

"Why don't I pass you over to Mom now and then I'll talk to you when she's finished."

"Karen? Hi, sweetie." Her voice was so faint.

"Hi Mom. Geordie's with me; we were just at the doctor's. We're having a boy! Your grandson's name will be Jeffrey Walker Young, after Mimi and Grandma Young's maiden names."

Tears ran down my face and I squeezed Geordie's hand.

I could tell that Mom was also crying as she answered.

"That's so wonderful. I'm passing you over to your dad so you can tell him yourself."

"Hi Dad. Your grandson's name is going to be Jeffrey Walker Young, after two of his great grandmothers' maiden names. What do you think?"

"I think that sounds terrific. That's just great. I'll let you talk to your mom a little more and then I'll call you later, if that's OK. Love you, gal."

"I love you too. Bye Dad." I waited for Mom to pick up again.

"Hi Mom. So, what do you think about having a little grandson?"

"I'm so excited, I'm speechless. A few of the Second Saturday ladies may come over later. Am I allowed to tell them?"

"You can tell whomever you want. He's your grandson."

"How special. And you're coming home tomorrow? Are you sure?"

"I'm positive. I can hardly wait to see you. Now I'm going to go so you can rest up before divulging the news about your grandson."

"Ok. I love you, sweetie."

"I love you too, Mom."

It was such a relief to finally know for sure that we were having a little boy, and to share his name with Mom. Geordie gave me a kiss and hopped in a cab to return to the office.

Aunt Cyndi sent out an email Tuesday night with an update on the day and all of the details she was handling in the event that Mom would be discharged on Wednesday. Once again, I was struck by how lucky we were to have such a strong family team taking care of Mom and each other.

Subject: Today's Update

Karen,

Here's a quick update of today …

Vicki has moved from W (Women's) 713 to W 715,
which is a private room. As Carole said today when she
visited, leave it up to Vicki to get a private room in the
penthouse. :)

She was more alert today than she was yesterday,
but she did have moments of confusion as well as …
increased difficulty breathing. The nurses talked to the
appropriate doctors, and scheduled a CAT scan for
tonight to rule out a pulmonary embolism, which could
prove fatal. At any rate, I believe she should remain in
the hospital unless they figure out what's wrong with
her breathing and determine how to fix it … It's always
something.

… I'll see you tomorrow. Have a safe trip and remember
to breathe.

Love you,
Aunt Cyndi

GOODBYE
March 2004

KAREN

Aunt Cyndi waved to me as I walked through customs at Washington Dulles on Wednesday. Her welcoming smile offset the resigned despair in her eyes.

She gave me a big hug,

"Hi, kiddo. I'm glad you're home."

"Hi, yourself. Thanks for coming to get me. Dad's at the hospital with Mom?"

"It looks like she is probably going to be released this afternoon, so we thought that made the most sense for me to pick you up so he can take care of her. I hope that's OK."

"Of course it is. I really appreciate it. Do you think we have time to run an errand on the way home?"

She gave me a conspiratorial smile. "Are you thinking flowers?"

We got home an hour later, laden with enough Osiana roses for flower arrangements in the powder room, kitchen and dining room, striving to make the house look special but not hospital or funeral-like. Aunt Cyndi watched as I walked into the dining room to see the hospital bed and other equipment she'd arranged. The bed was covered by a hand sewn quilt, pretty embroidered pillowcases and the multi-colored floral quilted pillow that one of their quilting friends had made. It was a lovely room to begin with and looked as inviting as a hospital bed setup can.

"Is it OK?" she asked.

"It's perfect. Thank you for doing this for her. She'll really appreciate it."

"Maybe. She might not be aware of it. But we'll know that it all is as it should be for her."

Just then, we heard the garage door open. Aunt Cyndi and I walked out as Dad was helping Mom into a wheel-chair. I leaned down to give her a hug and kiss on the cheek, then wheeled her up the two steps into our side door using the ramps Dad had made out of plywood.

Aunt Cyndi stayed over for a few minutes, and then went home so Mom and I could visit. I sat next to her on the sofa and held her hand. Occasionally, she gestured to the milkshake Dad had made her that was a foot away on the coffee table, and I reached over to get it for her so she could take sips through the straw.

"My doctor asked today whether I want to continue chemo, even though she as much as told me that she doesn't think I should have any more treatment." She bit her lip and took a breath before continuing. "I guess I should be grateful that she asked, at least. I need to decide what to do."

"Mom, I agree with her. I don't think you should have any more treatments."

She seemed taken aback by my quick response. I leaned in closer and held her hands as I continued with tears in my eyes. "You've endured so much treatment, for so long. You deserve to have some time to focus on yourself and your friends and family without chemo."

"Everyone's given up on me." She paused briefly as she gave into her tears, then switched gears before I could respond. "Sometime soon, we need to start talking about details. Not many people have four weeks to plan their own funerals."

"We'll start whenever you want to. I'll keep a pad of paper nearby to write things down as you mention them."

"OK, but not now, let's talk about my grandson now. Jeffrey Walker. I told the Second Saturday ladies his name; I hope you really don't mind."

"I'm glad you told them. What do they think?"

She perked up and sparkled as she responded. "What do you think? They think it's great, but of course they wouldn't tell me if they thought otherwise. How are you feeling?"

"I'm fine, just hungry as always. Dad's going to make hamburgers for dinner, but do you want a few crackers and cheese before? I'm going to get some for myself."

She ate one cracker with cheese. That, with half of her milkshake, four tiny bites of hamburger and a few small spoonfuls of baked beans made up her dinner. Soon after, Dad suggested they tuck her into the hospital bed.

"I'm glad you got that. I can't imagine trying to get upstairs to bed." Dad wheeled her to the freshly adorned dining room. She smiled and turned to me.

"It's so lovely. Did you do this?"

"Aunt Cyndi did it all. It really is wonderful, isn't it?"

"She's been just amazing through all of this. It must be so hard on her to be losing her sister. It's much harder for all of you than it is for me. I'm so sorry for putting you through this." She started crying again.

I didn't know what to say, so I just replied that I loved her and not to worry. I tucked her in with a kiss.

Dad slept on a foam mattress on the floor next to Mom's hospital bed all night. I was upstairs in the guest-room that used to be my brother's room. I stayed up for a while reading the book that Aunt Cyndi had recommended, written by two hospice nurses for caregivers helping as loved ones approached death. It was hard to imagine that we were close to this stage, but I hoped it would help me feel less floundering and more helpful with Mom.

Thursday morning, Dad and I met in the kitchen for breakfast. I asked him about Mom's oncologist's visit in the hospital.

"Even though she presented Mom with a choice, she clearly doesn't think she should continue with any treat-ment. She wants to see Mom again on Friday, to test her blood levels, but I'm not sure why else."

"Cliff? Karen?" We heard Mom calling us from the dining room and went in to greet her with smiles. Dad asked what she wanted for breakfast and made her a fried egg with a glass of orange juice. She sipped a little of the juice, and ignored the egg.

"I'd better be off. I love you ladies. Call if you need anything today."

"Bye, Dad." I gave him a hug.

"Could you help me to the sofa before you go?"

Dad reached down and slipped his arms under Mom's shoulders to hug her and gently lift her up with him. He shuffle-walked backward from the table to the sofa and eased her down. Then he gave her a tender hug and kiss.

"I love you so much." Mom and I were both crying as she responded that she loved him too.

After he walked out, we looked at each other's tearstained faces.

"We're a wreck," she chuckled.

I smiled, "Who, us?"

As I did the dishes, she slipped into a nap. I was sitting next to her when she woke up and very suddenly needed to go to the bathroom. When I put her arms over my shoulders and reached around her back to raise her to standing as Dad had done, I was taken aback to find myself bearing most of her weight. I felt the strain throughout my torso as I staggered backwards to ease her into the wheelchair, then onto the toilet and back to the wheelchair.

We decided to leave her in the wheelchair for a bit, as it wasn't too uncomfortable and it was clear that too much moving around wasn't great for either of us. She also conceded that she should probably use the rented commode from now on rather than trying to maneuver around in the confined powder room.

I was relieved that she'd made these two tough decisions herself since it was clear to me that I couldn't get her to the toilet again by myself. Not only did I nearly drop Mom, but I was worried that I might have hurt the baby. The next time she drifted off to sleep, I called Aunt Cyndi.

"Hi there, how are you?"

"Peachy keen and groovy," came her standard response. "How is everyone there this morning?"

"We're fine, but I have a question for you. You were going to come over this afternoon to meet the hospice nurse, right?"

"I'd like to, if that's OK."

"It's definitely OK. I was actually wondering if you could come over earlier."

I described what had happened and my concern about both Mom and my baby.

"I'm so sorry. I'd wanted to give you a break, but I don't think I can be here by myself with her."

"Don't worry, kiddo. I was looking for an excuse to come over earlier and you've given me the perfect one. I'll be over as soon as I can."

"Thank you." I was relieved and grateful when I hung up.

That afternoon, a hospice admissions nurse came and spoke to Mom, Aunt Cyndi, and me about various aspects of Mom's care. She told us about the full array of home hospice services, from the sponge baths she would arrange three days a week to pain management and any necessary equipment. She also gave us several numbers, including the 24-hour hospice help line.

She reinforced Mom's doctor's recommendation to let Mom eat only what she wanted, but not to force anything. I remembered reading in Aunt Cyndi's book that patients often stop eating as they approach death. It was another sign.

Dad got home late that afternoon just before the oxygen tank arrived. While Mom slept, Aunt Cyndi and I shared our concerns that two people be home with her at all times.

"When she needs help or attention, she needs it imme-diately and can't wait. One person alone hardly has time to go to the bathroom, much less prepare meals or deal with all the calls with hospice and Mom's friends."

I added, "And I'm afraid I'll hurt the baby if I lift her myself again."

Dad conceded, and reassured us that he'd be home anyway on Friday to help me take her to her oncologist appointment, and then it would be the weekend.

Mom woke up totally coherent on Friday. Even so, it took nearly an hour of joint effort for us to get her ready and in the car for her appointment. The nurses greeted us with hugs that seemed even kinder than usual. I could hardly stand it and couldn't imagine how they could bear to go through this with patient after patient. I already had the utmost respect for them, which grew during our final visit.

Mom only had one question during our visit, which she first asked the nurses and then her oncologist. Through her tears, she blurted, "Was Marilyn in pain? Was there a lot of pain?"

Both the nurses and her doctor assured her that Marilyn's death had been painless, and that hospice would take care of her so that she wouldn't feel any pain either.

Mom cried again as the nurses hugged her before we left. She started to say something about being here for the last time, and then retreated into her tears. I walked behind Dad as he pushed her wheelchair out of the office.

Mom was asleep when the social worker and hospice nurse came that afternoon. The nurse was armed with instructions for managing her pain with a combination of oral and intravenous narcotics, and her various anti-anxiety and depression medications. The nurse gave us a "comfort pack" for the refrigerator in case we needed anything else immediately over the weekend. I furiously took notes from her instructions for Mom's medications, and then second guessed myself as I read them over and over trying to memorize the suggested balance of medicines that were now Mom's only sustenance.

I kept scribbling as the nurse told us that the most likely next stage would be for Mom to become increasingly lethargic, and finally to go into a deeper and deeper sleep, leading to a coma and then her death. I hid behind my note taking, not allowing myself to think beyond the practical, logistical level of what I was hearing.

Drew and Lynda were there when Mom woke up on Saturday morning. She was so happy to see them, and kept saying that it was wonderful to have everyone together. She was hungrier than she had been and had a small glass of orange juice and half glass of milkshake, and even a few bites of chocolate doughnut.

After breakfast, Dad and I helped her through another urgent bathroom attempt. As she sat on the commode, she looked at us and said, "I wish this wasn't the end."

I bit my lip, and then replied, "We wish it wasn't too."

She looked at me gratefully and said that it was the nicest thing I could have said to her, leading us both to tears. Dad walked back to the kitchen and she commented that he wasn't crying. I suggested that the size of his tears was inversely proportional to his size, at which she gave a wry laugh.

We were all in new territory and it was so hard to say or do the "right" thing. Later that morning, Mom apologized for taking so much time to prepare for us to move her in bed and Drew gently told her that, "We have all the time in the world."

She burst out, "That's an awful thing to say. The one thing I don't have is time." Poor Drew looked like he'd been slapped and apologized as he fled the room.

After she settled back down, I went into the kitchen and put my hand on his shoulder.

"You know she didn't mean that, don't you?" He said that he understood, but I think my baby brother grew about five years older that morning.

Later that morning, the Second Saturday ladies arrived, laden with fruit, meals and calorie-laden pastries. Mom had a wonderful visit with them, chatting and joking. When Claire had to leave early, Mom said she wouldn't see her again. Claire replied that she would see her when she got back from her trip. Mom just shook her head. When Nancy, Jean, Carole, and Willie were ready to leave, Mom hugged them each in turn and exchanged a few words. I went to the foyer to let the ladies out, and they each gave me tearful hugs as they left.

That afternoon when Mom woke up from her nap and asked for Dad, I said he was paying bills. She responded, "I only have a week left; he can do that later." I called for him as I thought about how her perceived time remaining had shifted from four weeks to one in just a few days.

Dad, Drew, Lynda, and I gathered around her bed and she smiled gratefully to have us all there. She looked at Dad, who was wearing his work jeans and a tee-shirt and joked, "Since it's Saturday, I guess I have to let you wear your awful work clothes?" He shrugged sheepishly and offered to change, but she said no.

I gestured to Drew's John Deere cap and overalls and quipped that Drew hadn't felt the need to dress up either. Mom looked affectionately at her son and smiled, saying, "Don't ever change. I mean it, don't ever change."

She wanted to talk about "disposition of assets". This had become the only topic she seemed to care about and she asked both Drew and me which of her things we wanted to have. We talked a bit about who should get her jewelry and other things, because we all wanted to comply with her wishes. But I could tell that none of us cared about anything except that we were losing her.

By the time Aunt Cyndi and Eric arrived that evening, Mom was almost incoherent, in stark contrast to her witty, lucid conversations with the ladies and us earlier. Several times she mentioned that she was starving, but didn't want any of the food we offered her. Dad suggested that maybe she was saying that she was trying to starve.

I got up several times that night to go down and help Dad give Mom her pain medicine. She seemed to sleep pretty well, with only a couple of wakeful periods. On Sunday morning, I was in the kitchen when I heard a noise and Dad and I went in to see her. He tenderly adjusted her quilt and we noticed that the sheet she was laying on was soaked in blood.

The hospice nurse who arrived later that morning to check on Mom said that the blood indicated some type of "event", that indicated that she probably only had a few days left. She gave us new medicines to help Mom with the raspy, wet cough that had started to plague her breathing even further, and with the anxiety that had started to break through her standard medications.

I was in the kitchen writing up the new schedule of Mom's medications when Drew came in from the dining room with red-rimmed eyes.

"I just spent some time talking to Mom. This is probably a good time if you have anything you want to say to her. I think you should."

I wasn't ready. I took a deep breath. And another. Then I went in and held Mom's hand and talked to her. I told her how much I loved her and how lucky I was to have her as a role model to help me raise our kids the way she'd raised Drew and me. I described the reception we were planning for after her memorial service, reassuring her that everything would be tasteful and first-class. My tears flowed faster as I told her that we would miss her terribly, but that we would manage somehow and that she should leave us when the time was right for her. I promised her that Dad, Drew, Aunt Cyndi, and I would take care of each other and keep our family close, and that we'd tell her grandkids about their GG. I told her that I'd finish our book, even though I didn't have any idea how I would do so without her writing alongside me.

That night, Drew, Lynda, and I joined Dad on sleeping bags and mattresses on the living and dining room floor near the hospital bed. I was up most of the night, giving Mom her oral medications using a medicine dropper as she slept or stirred briefly. I called the 24-hour hospice line several times to confirm dosages and frequency, and wound up resorting to the comfort pack in the refrigerator to meet her needs until the pharmacy opened Monday morning. At nearly every minute of the night, either Dad and I or Drew and Lynda were by her side, so whenever she woke, she had us there caring for her.

In the middle of the night, she woke up asking for Willie.

"Where's Willie?" she asked, over and over. When we explained that Willie was at home, she asked, "Why is she home? I need to see her." We reassured her that Willie would be by in the morning.

Monday morning, I called Willie's house and told her husband that Mom had asked for her. Within the hour, he'd picked her up from work and brought her over for a visit. I was afraid that Mom wouldn't remember asking for Willie, but she was relieved to see her friend and they had an intimate, brief visit. While they were together, her husband confided to me that when Mom had said good bye to Willie on Saturday, Mom insisted that she would see her again. I was amazed that somehow Mom had anticipated her need for additional closure with this particular friend.

At the nurse's recommendation, we tried to limit unnecessary stimulation, keeping the lights dim, outside noises low, and sitting close enough to show our love, but without smothering her. She was never alone. Whenever she opened her eyes, she saw the face of someone she loved. Several times, she called for Dad or me, needing us urgently, so we made sure not to be more than a minute away at any time.

Mom's conscious moments were increasingly offset by an uneasy sleep. When she awoke, she made statements that sounded like preparation for her coming journey. She called several times for "Daddy", her father who had passed away when she was twenty-five, and "Jack", her brother with whom she'd reconciled and become friends a few years ago. She mentioned "my funeral", which we assured her we would handle as she would have wanted. Several times, she said to "take care" and we promised that we would take care of ourselves and each other.

At one point, she looked at Drew and Lynda and clearly told them, "I want a cup of coffee and I want it now." As they laughed, Drew ran into the kitchen to frantically cool down a small cup of coffee, which he offered her with a straw. She wisely declined it, but had made us all laugh with her demand.

Her repeated mantra toward the end of the day and into the night was a breathless, "Let's go, let's go, let's go." It really did seem that she was ready at last. She struggled to breathe and tossed and turned anxiously. I gave her the morphine as frequently as I'd been told I could, calling the hospice help line several times to ask about increasing the dosage. Aunt Cyndi and Eric had brought sleeping bags to join ours on the floor, though none of us slept for more than a few hours. Lynda stayed up most of the night singing softly to her. The exquisite voice of her loving daughter-in-law seemed to be the only thing that calmed Mom. As I drifted off for a bit of rest, I gratefully looked over to see Drew and Lynda beside her.

At about four o'clock in the morning, I couldn't stand hearing Mom's restlessness anymore and called hospice one last time to beg them to increase her dosages. I increased her intravenous morphine and after about an hour, she slipped into a comfortable, relaxed sleep. Dad and I sat next to her, as Drew and Lynda finally went to sleep themselves.

At seven o'clock, it was time for her next oral dose of medicine. As I put the first of two milliliters in her mouth, her throat made a gurgling sound and her breathing stopped. Dad and I looked at each other for a few long seconds, and then turned back to her as her breath caught again, even more sodden and labored than before. As I gave her the second milliliter she took her last breath. Dad gently squeezed her hand, and I kissed her forehead one last time.

That afternoon, I wrote my final update email.

Sent: March 16, 2004

Dear all,

I am sorry for sending a group email but I can't bear to write this one multiple times. After a courageous four and a half year struggle with ovarian cancer, fought every day with style and grace, my mother passed away this morning.

Her last days were spent with our family at home in Arlington surrounded by love. The worst lasted only a few days and her last hour was peaceful. We couldn't have imagined how difficult this day would be, but we knew it was coming and are comforted by knowing that she is no longer in pain. We were so lucky to have had our four "bonus" years and are trying to think about how fully she lived her too brief life.

Love, Karen

EPILOGUE
June 2011

KAREN

I have thought about my mother every single day in the
seven years since she left us. At first, my grief consumed and
depleted me. Sometimes it still does, as I face new adventures and challenges without her advice. More often, I smile
and think of her when I see something I want to show her,
or an idea to share with her or news that I know she'd be
delighted to hear. I wish she could visit us in our new home
in Toronto and drive with us to our cottage overlooking the
Restoule falls just down the hill from Geordie's parents.

Mostly, I wish she knew my children. I try to help them
know her through GG stories, which they love to hear.

I often say that Jeffrey's arrival saved me from my grief
at losing Mom. It has been a joy to watch him evolve over the
past seven years — from digging and building to Star Wars
LEGO and sports. He may not be the fastest runner on his
soccer team or skater on his hockey team, but he compen-
sates with tenacious effort, scoring his share of goals. He

has an affinity for predatory animals — his first lemonade stand raised $100 to help save sharks from poachers, and he recently announced that he is half-wolf. He is intensely creative, from building ships and dinosaurs to writing and illustrating stories. Perhaps he'll write a memoir himself one day.

My daughter, Kathryn Victoria, shares more than her GG's name. At four years old, she also shares her GG's passion for fashion, especially shoes. More often than not, she transforms herself into a Disney princess complete with glass slippers — I only wish Mom had been able to make her dresses. Her signature look is a bow holding back her exceptionally thick hair. She loves to dance, run, and jump and has endless stamina — after all; she needs to keep up with her brother. She is ardent in communicating what she wants — and what she doesn't — prompting Geordie to say that she is just like me. I am counting the years until she's old enough to join me for Afternoon Tea.

Drew and Lynda have two sons — Andrew is a year younger than Jeffrey and Adam is a year younger than Kathryn. Andrew's dimpled smile reminds me so much of my little brother as a boy that I can only imagine what Mom would say if she saw him. Apparently, Adam inherited my brother's independent spirit — amusing Dad no end as he watches Drew cope. Both boys had their stage débuts at Donk's before they could walk. Drew continues to be a pivotal influence for the kids in his community in his dual roles as the elementary school principal and award winning high school cross country coach.

My Aunt Cyndi's creative enterprise is booming. She shares her quilting gift with others through workshops and lectures while creating ever more innovative pieces for exhibition and sale. She is a repeat exhibitor, presenter, and teacher at Houston's prestigious International Quilt Festival. *Teal Beauty*, the tribute quilt she created — with the help of her quilting friends — to remember her sister, raised £4,500 for The Institute of Cancer Research at one of my "Breaking the Silence" events. In her free time, she moonlights as a communications consultant.

The Second Saturday ladies hosted a baby shower for me when I was back for Dad's birthday, less than a month after Mom passed away. We laughed and cried together as we shared memories of my mother. They've continued to be wonderful friends and mentors to me, and I was thrilled when they welcomed another woman into their group, so that once again there are six vibrant, energetic Second Saturday ladies.

After some long, lonely months, Dad found love again and was married in 2006. His wife, Judy, was once his high school girlfriend, with whom he was reacquainted forty-two years after he last saw her. She couldn't be more different from Mom, except for the two characteristics that are most important: she makes Dad happy, and he loves her. Judy's second grandchild was born on the day before what would have been Mom's 60th birthday. I believe that there's wonderful symmetry in that.

Kathryn was born on my final day as President of the Junior League of London. During my term, I grappled with many of the same issues that I remember Mom resolving for the Junior League of Northern Virginia. A few years ago, the Junior League of Northern Virginia decided to name one of their three membership awards after her. The Victoria Zacheis Greve award is given each year to an unsung hero, a woman who works behind the scenes to create huge impact with little recognition. Mom would have laughed at the oxymoron of being recognized for volunteering without recognition, but I hope she would be grateful for the honor.

Mom always said that among her many professional, volunteer, and other roles, her favorite jobs were those of wife and mother. I couldn't agree more, and know that my role as her daughter is the one that best prepared me to be a wife and mother myself.

Thank you, Mom. I love you so much.

ACKNOWLEDGEMENTS

This book tells the story of four and a half years in which my mother persevered with style and grace against the ovarian cancer that silently and insidiously threatened her life. I think of these as her "bonus years".

First and foremost, this book is dedicated to the doctors, nurses, researchers and other medical professionals who made these bonus years possible. Several of Mom's many doctors are characters in this book. We have not named you, as we wouldn't want our completely biased opinions to impact how others perceive you. You know who you are and we are forever grateful for the efforts that every single one of you made to keep my mother alive. Our heartfelt gratitude also goes to those scientists and doctors, mostly unknown to us, whose ground-breaking efforts created the myriad treatments that sustained her life.

Yet despite decades of innovative cancer research, my mother ultimately died because the treatments that could have saved her did not yet exist. For that reason, the profits of our story — should there be any — will be donated in support of cancer research.

There are several people whose support turned this book from idea into reality. To my former colleagues at Bain & Company, thank you for enabling me to make the leap from full-time consultant to part-time author. To Jo Parfitt, thank you for your editing advice that halved the length of this book and more than doubled its readability.

To Hilary, my friend and gifted designer, thank you for intuitively creating and perfecting our book's inspired cover and title and for meticulously laying out each page of our story.

To Aunt Cyndi, your final touches found many elusive typos and your thoughtful suggestions helped to ensure that our story would stand the test of time. But those are only the most recent of your contributions to this story. Thank you for willingly wearing so many hats since 1999, among them chauffeur, confidant, medical assistant, creator of fabric diversions and especially, with our love and greatest appreciation, sister, aunt, and friend.

To those whose love and friendship supported my mother throughout her cancer ordeal, and supported me then and since she passed away, thank you more than words can say. Mom once said that she hesitated to create a list, for fear of omitting someone. I agree, so this isn't a list but rather a few highlights. To the fabulous Second Saturday Ladies, Nancy especially, your friendship to my mother was without equal. To Victoria, Becky, and Anne-Marie, thank you for helping me be the daughter I needed to be without forgetting the person I am. To Lynda, your exquisite voice is second only to your steadfast loyalty and we are so happy that Drew brought you into our family. To Vivian, thank you for wisely, thoughtfully, and patiently being there for me until I was ready to embrace you as my second mother and my children's wonderful Nana.

Finally, for the men in our lives, Drew, Dad and Geordie, I find myself struggling for words. Ironically, I suspect that each of you may secretly wish I'd had writer's block a few years earlier. You are such private people and I am still amazed and grateful that you supported Mom and me in writing our story and now in sharing it with others.

To Drew, thank you for being there when our mom needed you, and for continuing to live a life that would make her so very proud of you. To Dad, Mom wrote her own words, "The best part of my life is Dad." Dad, I love you so much, for the father you are to me and for the husband you were to Mom for nearly four decades. To Geordie, Mom loved you and knew you were the best part of my life even before I did. Thank you for giving me precious weeks with her in Virginia while our lives were in London, and for giving me a reason to live when she was gone. You are my home and I love you.

ABOUT THE AUTHORS

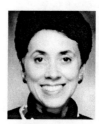 VICTORIA ZACHEIS GREVE was a dedicated volunteer serving the Washington, DC community for more than three decades. Vicki, as she was called, worked with a variety of nonprofits as an officer and board member and served as President of the Junior League of Northern Virginia, which posthumously named its award for distinguished service in her memory. After a 20-year "maternity leave", she managed taxes for nonprofit organizations for KPMG. She was the first in her family to go to university, graduating with a BS from the University of Delaware and with a Masters in Taxation from George Washington University. She was married for 36 years to her college sweetheart with whom she had two children. She passed away from ovarian cancer in March 2004, four months before the birth of her first grandchild. Her grandchildren love stories about their Grandma Greve, or "GG", a name she chose herself in eager anticipation.

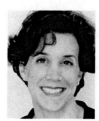 KAREN GREVE YOUNG is an American living in Toronto, Canada. She is a Past President of the Junior League of London and has served as a volunteer for the Institute of Cancer Research, the Junior League, and other nonprofits in Toronto, London, and San Francisco. Her work experience includes organizational strategy, management consulting, and finance. She has a BA from Harvard University and an MBA from Stanford University's Graduate School of Business. She is married with two young children. She misses her mother every single day.

343

CPSIA information can be obtained at www.ICGtesting.com
Printed in the USA
239159LV00005B/2/P